Praise for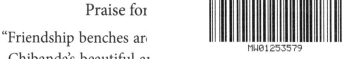

"Friendship benches are [...] Chibanda's beautiful an[...] [...] who reads it."

— **Johann Hari**, bestselling author of
Lost Connections and *Chasing the Scream*

"This is an amazing book. *The Friendship Bench* is a truly profound story of abandonment trauma and the healing power of connection: To be heard, to be acknowledged, to be anchored in a relationship of empathy is to begin healing our deepest wounds. It is so very moving to imagine the impact of these grandmothers creating connection with people who are hurting, and helping them heal with simple acts of love."

— **Susan Anderson**, bestselling author of
The Journey from Abandonment to Healing
and *Taming Your Outer Child*

"Loneliness, depression, mental illness, substance abuse — our world is desperate for solutions to these stubborn human plagues, and Dixon Chibanda is promoting a beautifully simple one. In my work reimagining midlife, I've seen the power of intergenerational connection and how the immense wisdom and value of our elders is often squandered. Chibanda has been doing extraordinary work leveraging this vital human resource, working with grandmothers to offer solace and direction to those who are suffering the worst. This wonderful book shows us that we don't have to rely only on professionals to help, that we are all each other's keepers, and that simple human connection can be the greatest cure. Read it — you'll love it!"

— **Chip Conley**, bestselling author of
Learning to Love Midlife

"This book is a marvel. As a practicing psychotherapist for four decades, I keep up with recent books about the field — they often introduce useful new ideas, techniques, and theories. I have not, however, read anything that has moved, enlightened, and excited me as much as Dixon Chibanda's *The Friendship Bench*, which is full of transformative wisdom. This book's time has come, and it contains lessons for those of us in the mental health field and for people looking for a new definition of eldership. I cannot recommend it highly enough."

— **Linda Carroll, LMFT, BCC**, author of
Love Cycles and *Love Skills*

The Friendship Bench

The Friendship Bench

How Fourteen Grandmothers
Inspired a Mental Health
Revolution

Dixon Chibanda, MD

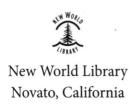

New World Library
Novato, California

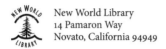

New World Library
14 Pamaron Way
Novato, California 94949

The stories in this book are true and the author has shared them as they were experienced
by him or by other characters in the book. Some names and identifying characteristics have
been changed to protect privacy.

The material in this book is intended for education. It is not meant to take the place of diagnosis and treatment by a qualified medical practitioner or therapist. No expressed or implied
guarantee of the effects of the use of the recommendations can be given nor liability taken.

Text design by Tona Pearce Myers
Photo credits: Pages xii, 24, 96, and 185: Costa the Creator / PictureHubZim.com; pages
72 and 114: Brent Stirton / Getty Images; page 130: African Mental Health Research Initiative (AMARI); page 148: Peter Nakhid, New Orleans; page 182: Jeffrey Prost-Greene
at HelpAge USA.

Library of Congress Cataloging-in-Publication data is available.

First printing, April 2025
ISBN 978-1-955831-02-4
Ebook ISBN 978-1-955831-03-1
Printed in Canada

10   9   8   7   6   5   4   3   2

New World Library is committed to protecting our natural environment. This book is made
of material from well-managed FSC®-certified forests and other controlled sources.

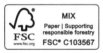

MIX
Paper | Supporting
responsible forestry
FSC® C103567

To the first fourteen,
who paved the way for thousands of others

Kukura kurerwa.
(Personal growth and wisdom are nurtured
by community elders.)
— Shona proverb

Welcome to Westfield Athenaeum!
A receipt of your transaction:

Original Balance:	$21.00
Payment Method:	Cash
Payment Received:	$21.00
Payment Applied:	$21.00
Billings Voided:	$0.00
Change Given:	$0.00
New Balance:	$0.00
Note:	

Specific Bills

Bill #	Lost	Received:
138849199	Materials	$21.00
37477007186486 Friendship bench : how fourteen grandmothers inspired a mental health revolution		

Contents

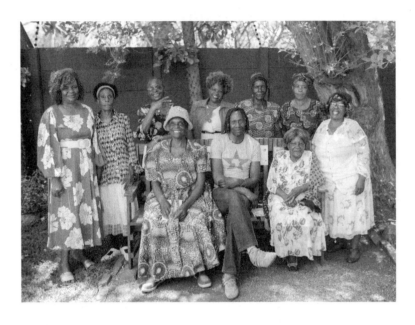

Celebrating the lives of the remaining grandmothers together with them in 2023. Standing from left: Shelly Tshimanga (aka Nurse Shelly, the first mental health supervisor I worked with), Monica Chizhande, Juliet Kusikwenyu (aka Grandmother Kusi), Felistas Gasa, Shelter Nhengo, Trader Karuma, Cecilia Mushambi. Seated from left: Marylee Chikwanha, me, and Sekesayi Hwiza. By the end of 2024 we had lost Monica and Marylee.

Preface

On a warm August morning in Harare, the capital of Zimbabwe, a twenty-four-year-old mother of two named Farai walked up to a park bench where an eighty-two-year-old woman known to the community as Grandmother Jack sat. Farai handed Grandma Jack an envelope, which the elder proceeded to open. After she quietly read its contents, Grandma Jack paused, took a deep breath, and said, "I'm here for you. Would you like to share your story with me?"

Tears poured down Farai's face as she looked at Grandma Jack. "I'm HIV positive," she revealed, her face filled with sorrow and shame. Grandmother Jack gently squeezed Farai's hand and, with not an ounce of pity in her eyes, assured the young woman, "It's OK to cry."

And with that, the malady that's known as *kufungisisa*, which roughly translates to "thinking too much" in the Shona language indigenous to the people of Zimbabwe, was lifted. Farai told Grandmother Jack her story, which set the wheels of healing in motion. All it took was a wise and empathetic person in the community to offer her undivided presence and attention, and from that moment onward, Farai's life began to change. She got a job at a local church, and with the help of her antiretroviral medication, the viral load in her body was substantially reduced.

During a weekly meeting of the Friendship Bench project, a community initiative started with fourteen grandmothers to address the scourge of mental illness, Grandmother Jack proudly shared that Farai had completely turned her life around: the troubled woman who had come to talk about her problems a few months earlier had transformed herself into a bastion of empowerment within her own community.

I'm happy to say that Farai was not the only person to have undergone such a paradigm-shifting experience. Over my years as a psychiatrist, I'd come to see that, just like Farai, people living with HIV and other medical conditions were more comfortable talking to grandmothers on a bench within their community than they were speaking to trained HIV counselors.

To this day, more than half a million people in Zimbabwe and across the world have benefited from the model of the Friendship Bench, which I created alongside fourteen dedicated, strong-willed grandmothers in 2006.

As one of only a handful of psychiatrists in Zimbabwe — a country of nearly seventeen million people that is still reeling from the impacts of colonization, war, poverty, disease, displacement, and other traumas that often remain unnamed and unaddressed — I recognized early in my career that mental health professionals were not sufficient to meet the needs of a struggling populace. This is true outside of my country, too.

On average, there is only one psychologist or psychiatrist

per 1.5 million people in underresourced parts of the world. In Zimbabwe, for example, when I started Friendship Bench, we had six practicing psychiatrists; today we have just under twenty. In Ghana, to give another example, there are just over thirty psychiatrists for a population of more than thirty-four million. Most of us are also aware that we are in the midst of an excruciating global mental health epidemic that has taken a harsh toll with respect to the sheer numbers of people living with depression, loneliness, anxiety, posttraumatic stress disorder, addiction, and suicidal ideation. In many parts of the world, adequate care is exorbitantly priced and out of reach for the average person.

I began this journey of creating the Friendship Bench in grief. Over time, I came to realize that while not everyone can see a mental health professional, most people have access to a vital untapped resource: the care, compassion, empathy, and wisdom of grandmothers — the unsung heroines of the world. Grandmothers weave together the fabric of community so that people's fears, their shame, and their loneliness might be alleviated, so they might realize that the burdens of life are never meant to be carried alone. Unfortunately, many societies do not value the contributions of the elderly as they should, but I am lucky to have been raised in Zimbabwe, a place that honors the unique leadership of those who've lived long lives and have the battle scars and profound awareness to show for it.

I know from firsthand experience that sitting with a grandmother who is listening to me with the utmost compassion while sharing her own vulnerability and humanity — as we talk beneath the trees on a wooden park bench in a safe space within the community — is far different from being in a crowded clinic, waiting to talk to a specialist who might only have a few minutes at most to assess my situation. And, of course, empathy and story sharing are seldom a part of the clinical process, as I knew all too well from my own work as a psychiatrist at a bustling hospital in Harare.

In the past decade, I have become more than convinced that the answers to the global mental health crisis do not lie in more diagnoses of disorders or prescriptions for medications. Opening minds and hearts to healing is possible only when ordinary people learn to support one another in extraordinary ways. Through the program of the Friendship Bench, everyday people have created healing communities that are learning to rebuild their lives from the wreckage of intergenerational and ongoing trauma.

In addition to one-on-one talk therapy with a grandmother trained as a lay psychotherapist, Friendship Bench clients who need more support are stewarded into a support group that we refer to as a Circle Kubatana Tose, or CKT. *Kubatana tose* translates as "holding hands together." In such a setting, community members empower themselves and one another to solve a range of problems, such as dealing with intimate partner violence or poverty.

Group members can relate to one another because they come from the same community and have learned the benefit of empathetic listening, in part through our training that specifically focuses on empathy as a tool for healing and in part through their own personal experience. This safe space in which to talk and be heard contributes to clients' sense of belonging and reduces the ubiquitous (but hopefully decreasing) stigma surrounding mental health and the sharing of personal stories. In the CKT groups, clients are also engaged in income-generating opportunities, such as vegetable gardening, bread baking, chicken rearing, and crocheting items out of recycled plastic and old VHS tapes. Not only does the group become a solid form of ongoing support; it is also a vital aspect of the mental health intervention, as socioeconomic distress is one of many determinants of mental health.

> *How ironic that we have been brought up to believe*
> *that we are poor when actually everything we need is*
> *right here in our community.*

— Lindiwe, CKT group member

One reason I decided to write this book, other than the fact that many of my colleagues and friends have urged me to tell my story for years, is that I want people to understand the powerful ways in which communities of individuals can make an impact by reaching out and connecting, especially across the intergenerational divide.

Although my story is mostly set in my home country of Zimbabwe, I have traveled the world and encountered many of the same problems in both developed and developing nations. Across the globe, we are beginning to recognize that the cultivation of community is crucial, especially given the number of people who struggle with loneliness and isolation. When we remember that we are not alone — that, in fact, we have priceless shared resources right under our noses, though we may not have seen them as such or even been encouraged to value their wisdom — transformation can happen. And oftentimes, that transformation can be life-changing.

Although many of us are in the practice of outsourcing our well-being and physical, mental, emotional, and spiritual care to institutions, such a tactic is not sustainable, because it's couched in a transactional and inherently limiting model. As human beings, we are relational. We relate to one another through shared stories and experiences. The value of a genuine smile, a warm embrace, collective laughter, and a kind word cannot be underestimated, especially in an era when our lives are becoming increasingly automated, atomized, and disconnected from nature.

I hope my story of the Friendship Bench provides an alternative to the somber stories that speak of the limitations of institutional healthcare settings. I want the world to recognize that a single person, no matter their background or level of formal education, can make a difference and play a pivotal role in their community. Each of us has a contribution to make that can result in the betterment of our community and our world — whether that looks like building a nonprofit organization, offering financial support to a worthy cause, or simply giving someone the gift of our presence and kind attention.

Of course, it took me time to learn these lessons. In working with the fourteen grandmothers who cofounded the Friendship Bench with me, I went through my own journey — from doubt and downright skepticism (I was, after all, coming from a theoretical, scientific research–based approach) to emotional breakthroughs I had not expected. I knew that I wanted to find a way to help the millions of people I would never be able to treat in a clinical setting, but I didn't know that the process of figuring out how to do so would transform me from the inside out.

I went from being a so-called expert to being a passionate

student who would continue to learn a great deal about humanity — my own and that of others — from the people I encountered along my path. I learned to embrace my vulnerability as an asset (although the field of psychiatry at large might beg to differ!) and to connect with people in ways that engendered genuine empathy, connection, and collaboration.

Throughout my journey, I've learned that storytelling is a profound vehicle for healing. The grandmothers I work with often use local indigenous idioms in recounting their own stories, which helps remove the stigma associated with sharing details about one's mental health (a stigma we are hoping to eradicate altogether). This has worked wonders when it comes to building trust, as we use a language and style people understand and can relate to. And, as we've found, magic is possible within communities where people can let down their guard, be themselves, and experience their intrinsic connection to the people around them.

We live in a world that tends to reduce complex human beings down to our component parts, a world that splinters us into discrete individuals and units. This keeps us from seeing the larger truth: that you can't observe one cell independent of another. We are all part of an intricate ecosystem of interconnected parts; if one part is unhealthy, the others inevitably also weaken.

My desire in starting the Friendship Bench was to help the people of Harare to work together to heal from four generations of trauma and to nourish a new way of being together.

The results of that intention are continuing to bear fruit, but as the grandmothers showed me, it truly takes a village for any meaningful change to take root and remain sustainable.

I never imagined that my little "village," which began with a cluster of fourteen grandmothers in a modest urban community, would become an umbrella for communities of people around the world who were eager to learn from our model. In November 2017, I gave a TED Talk about this work, which included aspects of my own story that I hadn't previously shared with a large audience. I never imagined that it would propel the Friendship Bench initiative to new heights and visibility around the globe. To date, millions of people have viewed my talk. Many of them have even traveled directly to Harare to meet and learn from the original grandmothers, as well as the more than two thousand grandmothers who subsequently came to be trained in our model so that they, too, could step up as leaders in their own neighborhoods and communities by providing support to people struggling with their mental health.

Over a decade of research, we've reimagined how evidence-based mental healthcare can be delivered. Instead of having patients arrive in a clinical environment where they are likely to be prescribed medication and sent away, the Friendship Bench initiative provides grandmothers with training as lay psychotherapists, as I mentioned earlier. We create safe spaces in the form of community-based benches (and now, a larger community center whose doors are open to the greater public) and offer group support based on collective problem-solving. This has resulted in an 80 percent reduction in depression and suicidal ideation and a 60 percent increase in clients' quality of life. My colleagues' and my seminal publication in the *Journal of the American Medical Association* in

2016, a cluster randomized controlled trial, showed that not only were grandmothers effective at alleviating symptoms of depression and anxiety, but after six months, 80 percent of clients who had sat down to chat with a grandmother on a wooden park bench were still symptom-free.

The value of the Friendship Bench far transcends statistics, however. The evidence that the model works is there for all to see, but what I hope to convey in this book is the reason why: we are each crucially important parts of a larger human story, and when we are gently, lovingly brought back into the fold of our community, we experience healing. I define *healing* as something that naturally arises when we are able to come together and be woven back into the greater whole. We simply cannot do it alone.

As someone who routinely felt alone in my occupation — an "expert" doling out prescriptions and advice to the less fortunate — my work with the Friendship Bench led me not only to a greater sense of purpose but to an awareness of my own belonging within a community of people who saw me as much more than the doctor with the authority to "fix" difficult situations. The grandmothers healed me, as well, by helping me to recognize and address the wounds I hadn't even realized I was carrying. They didn't do this with a prescription or any kind of conventional solution at all, but with the medicine of empathy and listening, which allowed me a space to grieve, to come home to myself, and to wholly dedicate myself to a process and a protocol that have the ability to save lives — something I know, because the process saved mine.

From the grandmothers, I learned that together we are greater than the sum of our parts. This is the core message of the book you have in your hands.

Every powerful movement in the history of the world has required people who are willing to gather around the proverbial campfire and generously share their time and energy with one another. So with that, I invite you to sit down and make yourself at home.

As you learn the story of the Friendship Bench, may you always remember that every one of us carries a powerful seed that is meant to grow and be shared for the betterment of our community and the world. I hope that my story and those of the brave women who were part of the creation of the Friendship Bench inspire you to do what you can to nurture your own seed so that it, too, may grow and flourish — so that the fruits of your efforts can be generously shared with others. My sincere wish is that all of us come to the understanding that while pain may be inevitable on this planet, so is healing. And somewhere in the world, there is a grandmother on a bench, beckoning you over with a welcoming smile — urging you to sit down, take a load off, and share what's in your mind and heart.

Chapter One

Erica

It was well after midnight when the phone rang in my house in Harare in March 2005. I struggled out of bed, groping along the dark passage toward the telephone in the hallway. Only the hospital ever phoned me on the landline. Through my grogginess, I surmised that it must be a new case; most likely, a junior doctor wasn't sure whether the drug they were thinking of administering was the right one or if the care they were offering was appropriate. They needed assistance from a more senior doctor, which was where I came in.

"Hallo," the female voice crackled on the other end. "Dr. Chibanda, this is the Baines Mutare Emergency Rooms. Please hold for the ER doctor."

A long pause ensued. Ordinarily, I wouldn't have been so concerned, but this was an ER at a hospital in Mutare, which was roughly two hundred miles away from the larger urban center of Harare, where I worked.

"Doctor?" This time it was the ER doctor, whose voice sounded faint through the static.

"Yes." I suddenly felt more alert.

"One of your patients is here, a twenty-six-year-old

female named Erica. She was under your care, and she's been admitted because she took an overdose of malaria tablets. It seems like it was a cry for help." He spent the next ten minutes narrating the circumstances that had led to Erica's deliberate act of self-harm. I listened, doing my best to gather all the pertinent details. My primary concern was what I could do next to ensure that something like this never happened again.

After he filled me in, we concluded that it would be best for Erica to be transferred to the state hospital where I worked. I would offer a full psychiatric evaluation as soon as she was well enough to leave the ER. Thankfully, her vital signs were already improving.

As I stumbled back to bed, I wondered how Erica's mother was dealing with this seemingly unexpected turn of events. I also recognized that the trek to Harare from Erica's rural village would not be easy for them. As I shut my eyes, I was struck by a twinge of concern…and some guilt. I had believed that Erica was making progress, but I also knew that deliberate self-harm was very common in Zimbabwe and was on the increase because of a series of intersecting factors that severely impacted the mental health of so many — especially our young people. Self-harm is not unusual in the face of strife and interpersonal upheaval, of which Erica had experienced a fair dose in the past few years.

The first time I saw Erica was in 2002, just after she'd turned twenty-three years old. She was training to become a primary school teacher. Erica was the youngest daughter of rural farmers who viewed her as their final hope for moving out of poverty, as her two older siblings had failed to make a decent living in professional careers. She had been a keen student in high school; naturally curious and intelligent, she received good grades and was now her aging parents' last chance at comfort and security. Naturally, Erica felt pressure to succeed, whether that expectation had been explicitly placed on her shoulders or not.

Erica's first bout of depression kicked in after she failed to attain the necessary grades to proceed to her second year of studies. She reluctantly resat for her exams, which was an extra financial burden for her parents, who were already struggling to feed the family against the backdrop of a severe drought. Her teacher training fees had been a massive investment for her parents, who relied on a small patch of land and six goats to sustain the entire family. They'd even sold their cow, one of their most valuable assets, to pay for her tuition the previous year.

When I saw Erica for the first time, we sat in my little consultation room, which doubled as a filing room at the psychiatric unit at Harare Central Hospital. Erica hunkered in a corner with a blank expression on her face, as her mother, Sekai, worriedly shared that her beloved daughter had stopped eating and talking and was now spending most of her time confined to her bedroom.

As far as social support was concerned, Erica had a few friends at the college where she studied, but Sekai was her primary pillar. Sekai told me that Erica had always been a playful, extroverted child, but after failing the teacher exam, her descent into depression had made her nearly unrecognizable. According to Sekai, Erica had stopped spending time in the mango tree where she often used to sit reading her books.

As it is for most people, Erica's decline was gradual. It began with self-imposed isolation; Erica spent more time in her room alone, although she came out occasionally to help her mother with cooking and other chores. Eventually, she stopped eating and frequently retreated to her room, offering monosyllabic responses to her parents' concerned inquiries. This carried on for a while, until Erica was referred to a general practitioner who put her on an antidepressant. Unfortunately, the dose, a measly 25 milligrams of amitriptyline, was not sufficient to treat her depression. On top of that, Erica suffered from side effects, including constipation, blurry vision, and dryness of the mouth. Her lack of interest in doing much of anything only worsened as she became more withdrawn.

"The general practitioner referred us to see a specialist," Sekai went on, sounding helpless. "There are no psychiatrists in Mutare, so we had to come here. It's a long bus drive — three hours."

I was sympathetic to her plight, but it was exhausting to consider the odds that were stacked against Erica. Like many of my patients, Erica came from a lower socioeconomic status than the people who frequented Zimbabwe's private hospitals. And at the government hospital where I worked, resources were scarce — which is why so many psychiatrists from Zimbabwe opted to leave the country for better opportunities. In fact, I was one of only six registered psychiatrists in Zimbabwe in 2005, which was challenging, given that we were then a country of twelve million people. (I'd studied in the Slovak Republic for my medical degree, but I had been eager to come home and contribute to my people's welfare. I naively believed that I could make a big difference if I worked in a large hospital. I ended up receiving a rude awakening regarding the power to make changes in any large institution over the course of my time at the hospital in Harare.)

I could sense Sekai's desperation; she wanted her child to be healthy and happy, but this would require a considerable sacrifice of time and money. I wanted to be able to come up with an immediate solution for Erica, but I also knew that rushing wouldn't lead to an optimal outcome. I also needed to consider treatment options. Moreover, I had to be realistic about what I could offer, especially because they might not be able to make the long trip to Harare for another two to three weeks.

Sekai cleared her throat, gazed at her daughter, and gently asked, "Can you tell the doctor what is bothering you, my child?" Erica remained tight-lipped, eyes fixed on the floor. Sekai sighed and turned to me again. She lowered her voice to a whisper, and tears flowed down her face. "Doctor, Erica was talking about ending her life."

I watched as Erica contemplated her sobbing mother. "Why are you crying?" Erica asked. As I observed Erica, I could see that her previous veneer of numbness was being replaced by genuine surprise, almost as if she couldn't understand Sekai's reaction.

"Why, my child, would you want to end your life?" Sekai sniffed as she looked forlornly at Erica.

Erica sighed miserably. "Life is meaningless," she responded, returning her gaze to the floor.

Silence filled the room, except for the birds chirping

outside in the guava tree. Their cheerful sound, which poured through the open windows, was a stark contrast to the mood inside the room.

I looked at Erica, who refused to make eye contact. "Was there ever a time when life was meaningful?" I gently queried.

Eyes still downcast, she replied, "When you anticipate that the next season will be better, life can be meaningful."

"Would you like to tell me more about that?"

The little finches in the guava tree got louder. As if she was waiting for the birds to quiet down, Erica took a long, deliberate breath. "When you realize everything is about the future and then, suddenly, there is no future…you lose hope."

"When did you realize there was no future?" I asked, straining to make my voice heard against the frantic crescendo in the guava tree. I could smell the ripe yellow fruit, which was abundant this season. The tree was paradise for the finches.

"When the seasons stopped to change," Erica responded, her soft voice a strange addition to the chorus. "It's like being in a hollow cave. I wake up and wish I wasn't there. I never used to have such thoughts. And I can't sleep. The tablets I got in Mutare make my mouth dry, and they also affect my eyes."

"Thankfully, that's something we can fix," I said, happy to provide this assurance, at the very least. "We can give you something else that won't cause those problems."

"Really? What would that be?"

"We could give you fluoxetine, but we need to find out what else is happening before we decide on medication." Although my work was clinical in nature and I routinely prescribed medication, there were other important protocols to be followed. I needed to understand Erica's struggle before I could determine the best way to proceed.

Erica suddenly looked up toward the window, startled by a commotion that was much louder than the finches in the guava tree. It was Resistance, one of our regular patients, exclaiming profanities at the male nurse, who held him by the hand as they walked past the guava tree toward the dispensary.

"That's a patient who is not doing very well at the moment, but he'll be fine," I reassured Erica and Sekai, who seemed a little alarmed. "He's probably going to talk to one of the other doctors. I'm sorry about the noise — today is really noisy all around!" I glanced at the guava tree and then back at Erica and Sekai to see if they'd prefer for the windows to be shut.

Erica shrugged. Sekai said, "It's fine, Doctor. You can keep them open."

I was heartened to see that Erica's curiosity had been piqued, meaning her eyes were no longer glued to the floor. Through the window, she watched as Resistance became increasingly agitated. "Is he mad?" she asked.

"No, he's just going through a rough patch."

"Am *I* mad, Doctor?" This time, she looked directly at me.

"No," I quickly responded. "But you need to tell me more about yourself before I can say what I think is happening, what we can do to help you, and if medication will make a difference."

"I wanted to be a teacher," Erica said glumly, with no affect whatsoever. "But I failed the exam."

"Doctor," Sekai promptly cut in, "we've told Erica she can still try again."

Erica sighed impatiently. "I'm getting old, and we don't have the money for me to try again."

I could tell that her mother wanted to intervene, but before she got the chance, a sharp knock sounded on the door. Nurse Takashinga stuck her head in and looked at us apologetically. "Very sorry for the inconvenience, Doctor, but can you please come and give Resistance his injection? He says he will take it only from you."

Resistance and I had forged a special relationship. He knew that I read the newspaper every morning, so we'd gotten into the habit of discussing the headlines and chatting about various topics. After I finished reading the paper, I would pass it on to him. I quickly learned that we wouldn't be able to proceed to anything related to his condition until I handed him the paper. Resistance loved speaking in a British-style English, using lots of big words to explain his points. This factored into his love of reading the newspaper and taking the time to explain the news of the day to me. He wanted me to give him the injection, not because I was a better doctor than any of my colleagues, but because our shared understanding had created a sense of trust.

I looked over at Erica and promised that I wouldn't be more than five minutes. As I walked through the passage to the injection room, I could see that the waiting room to my right was full; at least forty patients, many of whom had traveled from distant villages, sat in the hopes of being seen that same day. This was a common situation. I was the senior psychiatrist among a team of four; the other three were in training. Altogether we had our hands full with the clinic. I silently hoped we'd be able to attend to everyone within the next few hours.

The injection room was a tiny cubicle. Just as my consultation room had multiple purposes, the injection room also housed hospital files and acted as the dispensary. I walked in to meet Resistance, who was clearly distressed but well enough to acknowledge that he was relapsing because he had stopped taking his medication.

"What's happening, Resistance?" I asked, concerned but casual, so as not to elicit any further chaos.

"The voices are back." He shook his head. "Just give me the injection, Doctor."

"OK," I obliged. "I'm with another patient now, but I'm happy to have a chat with you later."

The nurse nodded at me. "He's being admitted now. You can see him after the clinic, Doctor. I know you have other patients to take care of."

I spent the next hour with Erica and her mother, doing my best to figure out how I could be of service. Her diagnosis was clear to me. She had all the symptoms of major depression: feelings of helplessness and hopelessness, poor sleep, withdrawal, a blunt and listless affect. I gave her a prescription of fluoxetine (also known as Prozac), and we agreed that she and Sekai would make the trip from Mutare to see me every two weeks.

After I said goodbye to them, I picked up Resistance's folder from the new admissions tray and wandered off to look for him. I found him slouched in an armchair in the recreation room, dressed in drab and depressing hospital garb. "Now, Resistance, why don't you tell me what's happening?"

"I just need a few days to rest," he responded. And then, predictably, "Do you have today's newspaper in your car?"

Resistance was in his late twenties and hailed from Mbare, the roughest neighborhood in town. This was his ninth admission in the past two years. The reason was always the same: non-compliance with his oral medication. I had never seen any of

Resistance's relatives in the three years I had been working at Harare Central Hospital. It was common knowledge among the staff that Resistance's father had died when he was still in junior high school. He had left Resistance a house and funds that were substantial enough to keep him going. At least according to Mbare standards, Resistance was well-to-do. But the lack of family and community support hardly made that privilege very meaningful.

Resistance was also the only patient I knew of who voluntarily admitted himself into this dismal facility. Everybody else was under Section 44, involuntary admission — and given half the chance, most would abscond. Resistance, however, seemed to find both purpose and community at the hospital. After the first day of admission, he would fall into his usual routine of assisting with chores around the facility, including cleaning and talking to new patients. He felt at home, accepted, free to be his full self here. Every staff member knew him, and all of us nonjudgmentally welcomed him back to the hospital each time he came in, swearing at the staff and demanding admission "because I'm psychotic," as he bluntly put it.

He always ordered an injection with each admission, and staff had learned to oblige to keep the peace — often just with a negligible dose or placebo. Over time, his mood became pleasant, even friendly. He enjoyed attending occupational therapy sessions and acting as a go-between for the patients and therapists. Ironically, his presence was stabilizing, as patients felt comfortable connecting with him, and he was reliable enough that staff could count on his assistance.

This had been Resistance's method of functioning for more than eight years; in many ways, he was part of the establishment. When a staff member fell ill and passed away, it was not unusual for Resistance to attend the funeral. He had become fond of the hospital, and we were fond of him. Here, unlike his experience beyond the hospital gates, Resistance thrived — most likely because he didn't face the same stigmatization and discrimination he was met with by his community in Mbare.

With Resistance, I'd come to understand the unspoken alliance that occurs between two human beings whose relationship is rooted in collaboration and respect. As a psychiatrist, I understood that my role was not merely clinical; it went much deeper than that. It rested on a basic understanding of our shared dignity. As the authority figure, I was not "better than" the patient, and the patient was not "less than" me. This recognition of our common humanity is the necessary ingredient in a successful doctor/patient relationship and for any kind of enduring treatment plan.

With Erica, it happened on her fifth visit.

Sekai sat in the corner, gently rocking in the wooden hospital chair, which was stamped with HCH (for Harare Central Hospital) in numerous places. This had been our attempt to discourage theft of government property, which never seemed to work. The HCH chairs could always be found in all sorts of places beyond the hospital, from hair salons to market stalls. Sometimes, the *C* was cleverly transformed into an *O* to read HOH, to disguise the fact that it was government property.

"Doctor, I think I'm ready to have our session without my mother in the room," Erica announced.

This is progress! I triumphantly thought to myself. We had established a therapeutic rapport that made Erica feel comfortable opening up to me. While I appreciated Sekai's commitment to her daughter's healing process — and it was always good to see patients accompanied by supportive relatives — I knew her ongoing presence might serve as a hindrance. Erica's mother was loving, but she was also controlling. Sometimes, in an attempt to move the conversation into a more constructive space, Sekai would interrupt Erica or discourage the expression of genuine emotions, like sadness. I sensed that Erica longed for the chance to shake off the "shoulds" and share her thoughts and emotions more candidly.

Predictably, Sekai didn't see the need. She looked at me, perplexed by the situation and expecting me to intervene. However, a split second of eye contact with Erica told me everything I needed to know — namely, that it was time to release her from her mother.

"So, Erica, would you like to have a one-on-one with me, without your mother?"

"Yes," she said.

Sekai grudgingly obliged and walked out of the tiny consultation room. Maybe she was wondering what family skeletons her daughter was about to dredge up.

"I love my mother, but I just think I need to talk without her today," Erica explained.

I nodded. "Of course. That's perfectly understandable."

She fidgeted in her chair, cleared her throat, and proceeded to stare listlessly at the ceiling as if she were searching for an opening, a place to begin. In situations like these, our most senior clinical psychologist, Dr. Alfred Chingono, would say, "Paying attention to the unspoken moments will tell you more about a person than their actual words."

I was contemplating Erica's long pause against the external background of nurses interacting with patients in the corridor when she began. "In our village, when I was growing up, there was a man called Tamba. He killed himself." She looked like she was trying to extract vital information about the past from the stained ceiling board. "His dead body…" She tilted her head, hunting for the right words. "He looked like he was just resting."

"Did you know him personally?" I asked.

"Yes. Everybody knew him. He used to fix houses. He was the best thatcher in the village. His house was along the road to school, so we would often see him as we walked to school."

"Is there a reason you're sharing Mr. Tamba's death with me?" I sensed that it was important for Erica to know that she was heard, but I wanted to cut to the chase, so to speak — especially since our session didn't afford us much time to linger on all the details. I wanted to understand how this story was related to her own mental condition and her reason for speaking to me without her mother present.

"It got me thinking about when I was suicidal. You know, when I first came here, I thought about dying a lot, and I always had flashbacks of Mr. Tamba's serene face…and I thought it must be OK."

"How do you know his face was serene?"

"Us kids saw him in the morning sitting against the wall of his house looking into the distance. We shouted, 'Good morning' like we always did, but he didn't respond. Then we walked into his yard. His eyes were wide open. He appeared to be looking through us, looking at something that was far away. I wasn't scared because he seemed so peaceful." Erica was now facing me, her face relaxed and comfortable as she spoke. "Interestingly, Doctor, right now I wouldn't want to die. Do you think it's the medication?"

"The medication helps, but talking is also very important."

"I actually sleep well now, and I feel a lot more rested. I don't spend most of my time ruminating and worrying about the future." She managed a smile before she changed the subject. "How is Resistance? Is he going to be OK?"

I smiled. "He's fine. He was discharged two weeks ago."

Erica's fascination with Resistance had been a running theme in our sessions. Once, when Erica came in for one of her reviews, Resistance was also present, so I had introduced them to each other. She'd greeted him with civility and respect, while Resistance was befuddled. "Who is this?" he'd queried.

"Just one of our patients who asks about you a lot, but always in a positive way," I reassured him.

Part of Erica's enthrallment had to do with his eccentric name. "Is he really called Resistance?" she would often inquire.

"Yes."

"That's so strange! Why would anyone give their child a name like that? Do you think something happened in his family?" It wasn't an unusual suggestion; in Zimbabwe, people normally get their names from specific events that leave an impact on the family.

"No idea. I've often wondered about that, too," I replied, realizing that none of us in the hospital had asked about the origin of Resistance's name.

I suspected that another reason for Erica's interest in Resistance was connected to any psychiatric hospital's association with conspicuous and severe mental illness. Often, people with anxiety or depression don't think they can receive help at such a place. I sensed that Erica was curious about how Resistance had become such an important presence at Harare Central Hospital; at the same time, she may have wanted furtive reassurance that she herself wasn't like Resistance.

I attempted to redirect the conversation back to Erica. "I would like to know more about how things have been at home now that you're back at teacher training school." Erica had decided to return to her coursework and prepare herself to take the exam a second time. I was hoping that she felt encouraged about her progress.

"I'm working hard again, Doctor. I'm a lot more positive about things."

"You certainly look more positive," I concurred.

"Thanks to you! I wonder, though, if we could cut down on my visits so I can just come in every other month. I know my mother will want me to keep coming every two weeks, but the truth is, we don't have the money for these bus journeys to Harare. If things become tough again, I can get in touch. But for now, I just want to focus on my studies."

It seemed like a reasonable request, yet I hesitated. "This makes sense, but do you mind if we discuss this with your mother, too? I want to make sure she feels calm about things when you head back home," I suggested.

Erica reluctantly agreed to discuss the issue with her mother present. As I'd expected, Sekai was not receptive to having her daughter cut back to a review every other month. Perhaps sensing the suggestion was based on their financial situation, she quickly offered, "We had a good harvest this year, so we're fine to come every second week."

"I don't want to come every second week," Erica insisted, her voice going up a register. In the end, we arrived at a truce: Erica would come in for review every other month, but we'd have a telephone call between visits.

We soon established a predictable routine. Sekai would call the hospital from a public telephone booth on a Thursday during my clinic hours to give me feedback on how Erica was doing. She'd then hand the phone to Erica, who always reassured me that she was fine. "My mother worries about everything and nothing," she'd say, laughing. "She should focus on taking care of her goats and garden while I study!" And always, she would blithely end the call with, "By the way, how is Resistance?"

While I'd harbored my own concerns about the infrequency of Erica's visits, she appeared to be doing well by most measures. During her hospital visits, Erica and Sekai always brought a gift from their garden as a token of appreciation for the staff: mangoes in season, a few cobs of fresh green mealies, oranges, lychees. Erica's mother would say, "I know you don't get paid much in a government hospital, and your services are free for us. Please accept these vegetables and fruits from our garden."

Some time after starting to work with Erica, I was honored with a short-term World Health Organization consultancy that took me to Benin for a regional workshop on mental health legislation and policy development. In retrospect, this was my way of exploring possible opportunities for work outside of Zimbabwe. Although I had initially felt committed to being of service to the people of my home country, I was beginning to consider what else was out there beyond the confines of Harare Central Hospital.

When I came back from Benin, word quickly got around that I had tasted some of the world's best pineapples in the city of Ouidah. During one of their visits, Sekai piped up, "Nurse Takashinga told me that you like pineapples. So instead of our regular vegetables and fruits, we brought you a pineapple!"

"That's very thoughtful of you," I remarked as I accepted the fruit, wondering if it would be comparable to the delicacies I'd sampled in Ouidah.

On a subsequent visit, Erica came in with more pineapples. "My mother wanted us to give you these because you love pineapples. As for me," she went on, smiling and placing her hand on her chest, "I love mangoes. I can spend the whole day in the mango tree in our garden eating straight from the tree! The mango tree is my second home; it's cool and peaceful and quite pleasant to climb up and sit there while I read my college books."

I liked imagining Erica sitting up in her mango tree, happily reading a book and gazing out onto creation. It heartened me to know she was experiencing more joy of late.

"You know something, Doctor?" Erica said. "I'm feeling confident about my studies — and most of all, after our chat from last time, I'm realizing that if I try my best, regardless of the outcome, I will probably not react impulsively."

"That's good to hear," I affirmed.

"It's been almost a year since I first saw you," Erica remarked as she gazed out the window. "The guava tree and the birds are back, so it must have been around this time." She smiled nostalgically.

Over the next two years, Erica's life transformed as she grew more at ease with her future while she prepared for her final exam. Because she was doing so well with her teacher training course and Sekai and I were both satisfied with the progress she'd made, I gradually weaned her off her medication. We also spent considerable time exploring a plan B in case her exams and results didn't work out. We decided that she'd become a teaching assistant as she prepared to take the test another time. A teaching assistant job would give her a modest salary, which would still make a difference to her family. With this plan in place, it seemed that Erica would be less likely, as she'd previously shared, to act impulsively. Even in the midst of another "failure," she would still have something to look forward to and work toward.

But when I received the call from the ER doctor in Mutare, it was difficult to rest easy about Erica. Despite three years of what had seemed like incredible progress on Erica's part, despite the trust and rapport we had established, despite the fact that things had seemed to be looking up, this turn of events shook my confidence. I didn't understand what had happened or why. I lay there in bed for several hours before falling into a restive sleep, unclear as to what my patient's future would be.

Three weeks passed after the call with the ER doctor in Mutare. It was midmorning at the hospital when Nurse Takashinga alerted me to respond to a call in the duty room. It was Erica's mother, Sekai.

"Doctor," she said in a muffled, somber tone, "Erica killed herself yesterday."

The world stood still. I struggled to make sense of her words, which were candid and final. I had been so caught up with work that I hadn't thought to call the ER in Mutare to check on Erica's progress. I felt the searing pain of remorse come upon me all of a sudden as I contemplated what I would have, should have, could have done.

"She hanged herself from the mango tree in the family garden," Sekai's voice echoed through the receiver.

"I'm so sorry…so, so sorry…" I could barely manage to get my words out. All I could think of was the joy that Erica had told me she experienced in the boughs of the mango tree. And now, the tree would always be associated with this terrible moment.

The silence that ensued seemed to last forever. Finally, I managed to say, "Erica was supposed to come for review as soon as she was discharged from the ER."

No sooner had I finished my sentence than Sekai cut in, her voice laced with bitter regret. "We couldn't make it because we had no bus fare to come to the hospital."

I felt the wetness of my palm around the plastic receiver, which I held tightly in my hand. Erica was gone…because her family didn't have money for a bus fare.

Sekai cleared her throat. "Erica had to stay at the hospital longer than expected to receive treatment. The hospital bill from the admission to the ER after Erica tried to kill herself left us financially crippled. We had to sell our goats to pay the medical fees because Erica ended up staying in the ER for a whole week."

It was a painful realization. I knew that Erica was particularly sensitive to the reality that her family had made many financial sacrifices along the way to ensure their daughter's success. The tragedy and cruelty of this simple fact was difficult to take in, because I surmised that guilt over being a burden to her family had led Erica to take her own life. The rest of the conversation was a blur, but when I hung up, I was left with a sense of my own ineptitude. After three years of what had seemed like an upward trajectory, I felt myself plummeting into despair.

Erica's suicide was a turning point in my career as a psychiatrist. I had found my calling out of a heartfelt desire to help the lowest echelons of my society — to offer solace where so few people found any. But now, everything was meaningless…the way Erica had said it was during our first meeting.

I had failed.

Nurse Takashinga, who was the longest-serving mental health nurse at the hospital, had seen it all before, so my despair didn't come as a surprise to her. She gently consoled me: "I know what you're thinking, Dr. Chibanda. But truly, there is very little you could have done in this case."

"I could have followed up…maybe called the ER to find out what had happened…" I trailed off.

She persisted. "And then what?"

"We could have facilitated an early admission. I could have sent them the bus fare to come to Harare." I shook my head. "It was only ten dollars. It shouldn't have been a limitation."

Her face was stern. "In 1995, we admitted Biggie Tembo." Biggie was a musician from the well-known Zimbabwean band the Bhundu Boys, whose contagious combination of rock 'n' roll, disco, country, and pop had made them a household staple. "He was suicidal, and we all knew it. I was on duty that evening. We knew he needed suicidal observation and needed to be in a safe place with nothing he could possibly use to harm himself." She paused. "He was in what we thought was a safe place. We were wrong. He hanged himself using his pajamas and the door handle. I contemplated resigning that same day."

She went on to say that despite her sorrow and guilt, she came to realize there was nothing she could have done. Certainly, miscalculations had been made about whether or not a safe space had actually been provided to Biggie, but a constellation of factors had led to his suicide; there was no single cause. It was a painful experience, but assigning blame was inaccurate and didn't solve anything.

Nurse Takashinga was close to my mother's age, and she'd been working in the psychiatric unit for nearly thirty years, meaning she'd seen it all. She had been especially helpful when it came to advising me on how to manage Resistance during my first contact with him.

"He's harmless," she'd reassured me. "He's just a very lonely man who needs to interact with people." I usually appreciated Nurse Takashinga's kindness and knowledge, and I took comfort in her wise counsel, especially in those moments when I felt frustrated and at a loss for words. Unfortunately, this was not one of those times. I could understand what she was saying about client suicides, at least intellectually, but as images of the past three years of working with Erica flashed in my mind — her playful inquiries about Resistance, her stories about spending entire days in the mango tree, her hope that she'd found a new way to deal with her problems — it was hard to accept that there was *nothing* I could have done.

The pain of this loss would linger for a very long time, and relief would come much later…in an unexpected form.

The acute shock of Erica's death gradually subsided at the hospital, and soon it was business as usual among the other staff; in contrast, I continued to struggle. Perhaps the fact that Erica and I had established a solid and trusting relationship was part of what made it so hard for me to accept her death. If I'd mistakenly believed she was on a positive trajectory, where had I gone wrong? Was I simply part of a broken system that placed Band-Aids on people's wounds without addressing the root causes? Haunted by guilt and impostor syndrome, I began to question everything, including the time-honored clinical approach to which all psychiatrists are bound.

Although I didn't immediately voice my concerns, which were gathering strength inside me in subtle and invisible ways, a new question haunted me alongside my memory of Erica: *Who else would have to die before we found a better way to address mental health struggles?*

For many months after her death, I thought of Erica's sense of humor, as well as the misty-eyed state she'd often move into whenever she discussed her dreams of changing the world, or when she talked about the young man she had gradually grown fond of, or when she shared her private moments of joy in the mango tree. I wistfully imagined Erica creating a space just for herself within the boughs of the tree so she could watch the clouds float through the blue sky while she contemplated what her future life as a teacher would be like. In my mind's eye, I could see Erica flying out of the tree and soaring into a different reality — one where everything worked out and there were many more good days than bad ones.

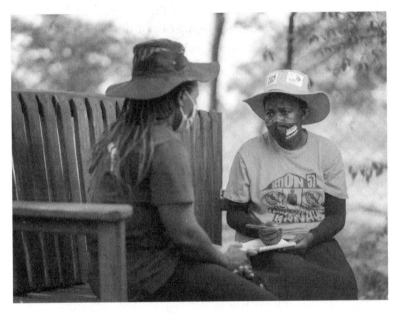

A grandmother conducting a session during the Covid-19 lock-down. We continued the program during the pandemic as the grandmothers didn't want to stop. All sessions were held out-doors, and we made masking mandatory. Fortunately, we didn't lose anyone to Covid.

Chapter Two

All of Us Are Vulnerable

I'd never really questioned my work as a psychiatrist, but now I was doubting it every day.

Prior to Erica's death, I'd simply been doing what everyone else in my field was doing: prescribing medication and taking a biological approach to treatment. Sometimes, depending on their symptoms and the assessment I'd made, I might recommend talk therapy within the occupational therapy department; however, ultimately, the emphasis was not on talking through the client's problems but on quickly identifying the solution, which mainly came in the form of a prescription. It was just the way I'd been trained. After everything that had transpired with Erica, however, I had a gradually dawning realization that it wasn't enough to simply offer medication. People needed something more, but I didn't yet know what that was.

As I pondered a possible direction forward, I was also dealing with some of the larger issues impacting Zimbabwe and its people. If you aren't familiar with Zimbabwe, it's vital to understand that against all odds, despite the challenges we face, including a potable water crisis and a bleak economic outlook, we continue to have a fairly functional primary healthcare system. The process of being referred to a specialist works smoothly. Other innovations that have made a difference and continue to improve Zimbabweans' quality of life include groundbreaking work around HIV/AIDS, a national immunization program, and strong maternal and child healthcare.

Unfortunately, many of the negatives can seem to outweigh the positives. Zimbabwe is a nation that has suffered four generations of trauma beginning with colonialism in the nineteenth century, when the British diamond tycoon Cecil Rhodes and his British South Africa Company started to infiltrate the area that was then known as Matabeleland. Two prominent spiritual leaders, Nehanda Charwe Nyakasikana (or Mbuya Nehanda, as she is more commonly known) and Sekuru Kaguvi, led the revolt against the British South Africa Company in Matabeleland before being hanged and decapitated. After Rhodes swindled mining rights from the Ndebele people and the region became a British colony, the Crown renamed it Southern Rhodesia. The effects of these events reverberated throughout the next century and gave way to the Rhodesian Bush War in the 1960s and the massacre of the Ndebele people in the 1980s.

I still recall my late grandmother saying she'd love to go back to her original land, prior to White people settling the region. She passed away before President Robert Mugabe oversaw a huge land redistribution initiative in the early 2000s. Ironically, this land redistribution, which was rooted in the seemingly noble cause of giving land to the people who needed it most and who had been stripped of their rights during colonization, was really more of a land grab and ended up causing greater harm than good. Unfortunately, the violence didn't end there.

On August 24, 2005, five months after Erica's suicide, United Nations Secretary-General Kofi Annan issued a statement about the destruction that had recently engulfed Zimbabwe. It was during June of that year that uniformed forces set out to systematically demolish every house and building across the country that had been deemed an "illegal structure" according to Zimbabwe's bylaws. It was a well-orchestrated initiative meant to quash the ruling party's opposition in primarily urban areas. This movement was known as Murambatsvina, which literally means "remove the filth" in the local Shona language. It was deemed a "cleanup" by the government, but it was much more than that. While the "cleanup" purported to eradicate slums and illegal housing that were hotbeds of disease and crime, the communities of low-income people, where the majority of the opposition resided, were demolished in the process.

I was a firsthand witness to the suffering of many displaced people as I drove to work each morning, but I myself was removed from what was occurring. Similar to South Africa, Zimbabwe had its own version of apartheid. Black people, Asians, mixed-race people, and Whites were segregated in their own communities. High-income areas of Harare and the nation at large were not affected at all. As in most parts of the world, it was the people with the least resources who suffered the most.

My work gave me much insight into the pain Zimbabweans had faced as a result of numerous senseless, ill-conceived initiatives that were motivated by greed and political gain. By the time Murambatsvina occurred, Zimbabwe wore the battle scars (and still-gaping wounds) of four generations of trauma that had never seen any true resolution. This had left the population on edge; it took just a little push for the tragedy to become explicitly manifest as a crisis of public mental health. Murambatsvina was a continuation of a predictable chain of events that had caused understandable animosity and resentment.

Trauma breeds trauma, and when we fail to create space for healing, it proliferates to create even more trauma. And it's crucial to note that Zimbabwe's story is not unique. The path to freedom in nations that have experienced colonization and genocide, including Australia and the United States, is fraught with challenges.

Together, many of the crises my country faced would gradually help me to realize where my efforts had to be focused and how I could honor Erica after her death.

Operation Murambatsvina was well into its third month when I received a handwritten referral from the internal medicine team at my hospital; it was about a young mother who had deliberately ingested rat poison in an attempt to end her life. The referral, probably written by a junior doctor, was brief: "Kindly see the above-named 22-year-old mother of one who fed her infant son porridge laced with rat poison before ingesting some herself. Her son did not make it. She is in the medical ward C5. She will need psychiatric evaluation."

When I got to C5, I was directed to a petite woman who lay flat on the bed with a nasogastric tube down her nose, connected to a breathing device. Next to the bed sat an elderly couple whom the nurse in charge introduced as the patient's parents. The father held his daughter's hand as she labored to breathe through the tube.

"Not much we can do with her in her current state," I said to the nurse. "Maybe I can get some collateral history from the parents if possible? I can always come back when she's up and able to talk."

The patient's mother, whose waist was wrapped in a traditional cloth, explained how they had to rush to Harare from their rural home when they'd heard their daughter had taken rat poison. "Her house was demolished a month ago during Murambatsvina," she whispered.

"She had nowhere else to go," added the father. "She stayed a few weeks with friends, but when nobody could put her up any longer…" He broke down weeping as he held his daughter's lifeless hand against his face. "She could have come home to the village, but she chose not to."

"Instead, when it was too much," the mother went on, "she went to the Mukuvisi River in Mbare with her three-month-old son and took poison." Her voice caught in her throat before she added, "He was our first grandchild."

I listened to the story, took down as much collateral history as I could, and promised to come back once their daughter was up and the tube was removed.

Four days later, I received a brief note from the nurse in charge in ward C5 saying there was no need to come back. The young woman hadn't made it.

The siege lasted just a few months, but the damage was done: by the time Murambatsvina was over, seven hundred thousand people were homeless, and an estimated two million had been psychologically impacted. This meant that a large portion of the nation's populace were dealing with posttraumatic stress disorder, depression, anxiety, addiction, deliberate self-harm, and suicidal ideation. In fact, at my hospital, I witnessed a surge in patients with symptoms of all of the above. We had been plunged collectively into a national crisis, and the only way out was through.

Witnessing the senseless suffering everywhere around me was overwhelming. I felt helpless in the face of all that was occurring. Many of the episodes of suicide and deliberate self-harm I was encountering were clearly linked to larger social determinants of health, including intimate partner violence, living with HIV, and the inability to access needed medication. As a psychiatrist, I had been taught that any kind of self-harm is a reflection of poor coping strategies. But if you lived in a place where you had no support at all, which was certainly the case in the aftermath of Murambatsvina, what then? It seemed obvious to me that people would resort to drastic measures.

The final report on the wanton destruction of homes was damning against a government that was still trying to recover from the poorly conceived land redistribution program, which had amounted to farm invasions. In Shona, these invasions were known as *hondo yeminda*, which means "the war to liberate arable land."

The invasions under Mugabe had begun in the early 2000s, when armed gangs attacked and took over White-owned farms. At the time, about 80 percent of the country's farmland belonged to a few thousand White farmers. This had been true since the 1950s or so, when the White farmers inherited huge tracts that had been stolen from Black farmers and given to the original European settlers who came to Zimbabwe during the earlier colonization period. The Black people whose lands were stolen were forced to live on tribal trust lands.

As I mentioned, my grandmother often talked about her longing to return "home," which would never happen. Black people had occupied fertile African land for centuries — very likely, millennia. They had learned which regions were conducive to production, and colonization took that away. The colonial process of land seizure was blatantly motivated by racism and greed. Not only were Black people robbed of their homes, their businesses, and their sense of a continuous relationship with the land, but after the establishment of tribal trust lands in 1930, they were eventually forced into even smaller refugee camps in areas with little arable soil for agriculture. And they could not leave.

I remembered being with my mother when we visited my paternal grandmother at one of those camps just outside our village of Murewa during the final years of the war of liberation, around 1979. The camps were referred to as *khips* in the local language; in Shona, this is a bastardized version of an idea that roughly translates as "being kept against one's will," which was entirely accurate. A khip was a square, upright thatched structure approximately five by five meters (about sixteen by sixteen feet) in size, without a roof. Seeing my grandmother being forced to live in a structure without a roof was the height of dehumanization. And she never stopped talking about it.

The Rhodesian forces made the structures roofless so they could see inside each house from their helicopters as they scoured the terrain for the so-called terrorists — Black freedom fighters who had been trained in Zambia and Mozambique, countries that had recently gained their independence from colonizing forces. The war was in its last stretch, and I was still too young to be considered a *mujibha* (an errand boy for the terrorists), so I was allowed to go to the village without any interference.

One evening we were all quietly reading the Bible in the candlelight just before bedtime. As I gazed up at the night sky with its innumerable stars, the adults all froze. It took me a while to decipher the distant sound of a helicopter. As the *tra-ta-ta-ta* got louder, my grandmother blew the candle out and held me close. I knew that something was wrong. There was utter silence except for the approaching roar. As the helicopter neared, it shined a bright spotlight down into each exposed khip.

When the light hit us, my grandmother held me even more tightly. I could hear her heart thumping against my ears. A voice echoed through a loudspeaker, but my head was too firmly squeezed against my grandmother's body for me to comprehend what was happening. The helicopter moved on, and the rattling sound faded into the distance. Even after the helicopter had disappeared and the only sound left was that of the night creatures and crickets (not to mention the thumping of my grandmother's heart), the silence among the adults felt deafening.

I learned a new lesson that night: deep silence is quite loud when it's associated with fear.

It was a difficult situation that I didn't fully understand until I was much older. To add insult to injury, many of the people who'd been displaced and sent to the khips had been forced to flee the areas where their families had been buried for generations. Culturally, one of the greatest violations imaginable for us was that of being removed from the resting place of our ancestors. Land was connected to identity in powerful ways that the White settlers neither understood nor respected. The way I saw it, much of the resulting fury and destructiveness had as much to do with seeing new buildings erected on the graves of Black people's ancestors as with the deplorable living conditions into which Black people were forced.

Strained race relations, and the bitter blood that remained, had made it difficult for Black and White people to peacefully coexist. During colonization, a White minority had instituted racist policies in almost every arena of public life. Although Black national liberation groups steered armed struggles against the White government in the 1960s and '70s, ultimately leading to a peace accord and Zimbabwe's independence, the White settlers' economic power had not been shaken.

While Mugabe's government had been amenable to White people in the 1980s, that changed during the farm invasions of the early 2000s. Violence was now encouraged against White Zimbabweans, and the racial discord was amplified to a whole new level.

Unfortunately, while the land seizures had begun as a way to ensure equitable redistribution to poor Black people, they quickly spiraled into a massive invasion that resulted in looting, destruction, and killings. It was yet another disaster that left thousands of people emotionally and psychologically wounded. Overall, the Zimbabwe Human Rights Forum reported, at least ten thousand people were displaced. While some people benefited, most did not. In the end, most of the land was seized by the elite Black political class.

The process had been too recklessly implemented — and, ironically, the primary driver was greed, the very thing that had forced Black people out of their homes during colonization. While extensive documentation, including legal injunctions representing more than a thousand White farmers who lost land, are available in the public domain, little is known about the approximately hundred thousand Black farmworkers who lost their livelihoods and accommodations during the period of madness that turned Zimbabwe from a thriving breadbasket into the region's basket case. Before the farm invasions, the nation had exported food throughout the region, but that was no more. Zimbabwe was now dependent on other nations for its food sources.

After Erica's suicide, many of the patients I encountered, including the twenty-two-year-old woman who had taken her son's life and her own out of sheer desperation, led me to more deeply consider that mental health wasn't merely about individuals responding to the circumstances of their lives in functional or dysfunctional ways. It was about the ways in which entire communities did or did not have access to healing. And with so many of the traumatic events that had occurred in the wake of colonization, wars, and the misguided attempts to make everything that had been torn apart whole once more, it was little wonder that so many people were suffering, with seemingly no way out. As I pondered the bigger picture, I also remembered that the struggle was not limited only to people like Erica.

One of the highest rates of suicide and substance use in Zimbabwe is among the White community who lost their farms during Mugabe's land grabs. I recollected that Koos Von Tonder was one of those people; he came to me in 2005, before Murambatsvina was laying waste to urban areas. He had agreed to see me only because his wife, Betty, threatened to leave him if he didn't.

During the Rhodesian Bush War of the 1960s and '70s, Koos had been a Selous Scout. The Selous Scouts were a special forces unit of the Rhodesian Army who focused on infiltrating the Black majority population and waging attacks on insurgents. My grandmother had often shared stories about the Selous Scouts and how ruthless they were when they visited a village suspected of harboring "terrorists."

Like so many others, Koos kept the trauma of war to himself. After 1980, he was among a hundred thousand White

Zimbabweans who emerged from the Bush War relatively unscathed — or so we were led to believe. He was only one of a few thousand White Zimbabweans who decided to stay after independence. Before Zimbabwe's independence, roughly 10 percent of the country's population was White. Now, it was probably closer to 6 percent or less. Many people had left, perhaps out of fear of retribution. Colonization had left a bitter taste in everyone's mouth.

Koos had inherited land just outside Harare from his father and became a successful commercial farmer, contributing significantly to Zimbabwe's export of fresh produce to the European Union. However, he was one among many who lost his farm in 2003, and the ensuing years were fraught with financial and emotional difficulty.

Koos and Betty drove 200 kilometers (about 125 miles) to see me, just like Erica, because there were no psychiatrists where they lived. As a White man, he was an unusual patient; most of the people who came into the hospital were Black. In our first session, Koos sat quietly next to his wife as he struggled to articulate his pain. "My farm was the best in the whole district," he softly said as he put his hands together — hands that were calloused and rugged from toiling under the African sun for decades. "I had a school, a health clinic, and accommodations with electricity and running water for all my staff. I paid the university fees for my staff's kids." He looked me in the eyes as his own began to fill with tears, which he fought back with a hard sniffle as he roughly brushed his hand across his face. "But my staff woke up one morning and turned against me. They betrayed me after all I had done for them. Why?"

As I always tried to do with my patients, I listened with

compassion rather than confirming or denying their subjective experience. I could see that Koos was in pain — and also that he hadn't thought about the larger historical context against which the land grabs had occurred. In his mind, the land unequivocally belonged to him — after all, he was the one who'd built the infrastructure of the farm from scratch — and it had been forcefully stolen from him. In his eyes, he was the only victim — not the Black people, like my grandmother, whose lands had been seized over decades of colonization.

Koos was a typical Afrikaner type: a large, burly, sunburned man with massive arms. He was the very symbol of the White man who'd come to Africa to conquer it, strong and in charge. But his words and eyes told a different story. Koos was fighting to suppress his emotions, which still managed to break through; I could plainly see the anger and grief etched into his face.

Betty tightly gripped his hand and said, "It's been a terrible time, Doctor. We lost everything." Then, turning to her husband, she gently nudged him. "But Koos, you need to tell the doctor about your drinking. That's why we're here."

Koos looked at Betty with contempt, lost in his bitterness. "A shit government!" He walked out, adamant that he didn't need to see a psychiatrist and didn't have a drinking problem. Shortly after this, Betty called to inform me that Koos wanted a prescription for a medication that could calm him down, which might appease his drinking problem. Of course, it was difficult to figure out what to prescribe over the phone, but I decided to start him out on a low dose of antianxiety medication, which I hoped would help.

Koos wasn't the only person I saw who was struggling in the aftermath of the land grabs. Many people were still dealing with the repercussions of much older, yet still relevant, national wounds.

Around the time I met Koos, I was paid a visit by a woman named Sibongile, who held her grandmother, Gogo Ncube, by the hand as she shuffled into my consultation room. It was the usual story: they had traveled all the way from Bulawayo, some 400 kilometers (nearly 250 miles) away, because Gogo Ncube needed a specialist who would help to address her PTSD and the visions that continued to haunt her into old age.

When Gogo Ncube spoke, she firmly held onto her walking stick. She hailed from the Silobela region of Matabeleland, an area that had witnessed some of the worst killings during the massacres known as Gukurahundi, which took place in the 1980s. It was nothing short of a genocide. *Gukurahundi* is a Shona term that translates to "the early rain that washes away the chaff before the spring rains."

Right before this terrible chapter of history, two rival factions of the Black nationalist party had emerged: Mugabe's Zimbabwe African National Union, which recruited primarily Shona people (the majority population), and Joshua Nkomo's Zimbabwe African People's Union, which was supported by the minority Ndebele and Kalanga peoples. Mugabe's party attacked dissidents in the Matabeleland South Province, forcing thousands of Ndebele and Kalanga into reeducation camps; others were tortured and executed. It's believed that over twenty thousand people were killed, but Mugabe's regime never took responsibility. Rather, Mugabe strengthened his hold on Zimbabwe by offering more support to the former freedom fighters who had fought against the White people. And, as we already know, Mugabe eventually gave some of these people authority to grab the land back from White farmers, which led to the nationwide breakdown of the rule of law.

"They came," said Gogo Ncube with a slight tremor while she recounted the horrific events of Gukurahundi. "They rounded us up. They put the men in a hut, closed it, and set it on fire."

Sibongile sat next to her eighty-two-year-old grandmother, wearing an indifferent expression. I knew it wasn't because she didn't care; it's just that she'd heard this story many times already.

Gogo Ncube continued, her eyes almost glazed over as she relived a period of history many would prefer to forget. "The young women were raped in front of us. Some were bayoneted. I have not stopped seeing those visions."

I sat in silence as her words lingered in the air. It was a problem that could not be solved by medication alone. After a while, Sibongile spoke. "Doctor, can you stop these thoughts and constant repetition about these events? All of us have been affected. Why has Grandma not moved on?" By now, the stony expression on her face had given way to tears and desperate sobs.

Gogo Ncube gazed evenly into her granddaughter's eyes and simply said, "How can I move on when I have the ghosts of my entire village crying out for justice?"

Her question remained with me for weeks. I wondered what justice would look like for a country of people who had suffered so much in the past several decades. Who would be held responsible? How could we tell the stories of millions of people from all sides who were still living with the trauma that had been inflicted upon them or that they had visited on their neighbors? Where and when would the cycle end?

One day in early October, just before the first rains, Koos's wife, Betty, called to inform me that her husband had taken his own life. It was then that I came to a somber realization: if Koos had lost his private battle with grief, all of us were vulnerable.

In the wake of Erica's death, as I remembered the patients who'd walked through my doors — Koos, the distraught young mother, Gogo Ncube — I felt that all my unanswered questions and silent anxieties had come to a head. Indeed, all of us *were* vulnerable.

When exposed to a specific kind of stress, in a sufficient amount and during a difficult time, any human being will break. Koos had broken because there was no safety net to protect him anymore. And in many ways, even before the land grabs, that safety net had never truly existed for other, much less privileged Zimbabweans.

With everything I'd witnessed in the past year and with the pressure that had descended onto my shoulders since Erica's death, I was beginning to recognize that perhaps the scope of my work was much larger than I'd initially believed. It went far beyond prescribing medication. It had to.

Chapter Three

The First Step — Opening the Mind

With the loss of Erica still lingering in the background, Murambatsvina proved to be the impetus for my escape, albeit partial, from Harare Central Hospital. In essence, I was running away from my failure. My encounter with Gogo Ncube had especially touched me, as I understood that the events of the past several months were part of a chain of tragedies in which too many Zimbabweans were also complicit. Although I myself had not perpetrated any of the violence, I hailed from the Shona, the ethnic group responsible for killing the Ndebele and Kalanga residents of Matabeleland. In some way, I felt the need for righting the egregious wrongs that had been done.

The horrors were not exclusive to the ones people had visited upon one another. They were also inherent in the harm that people perpetuated on themselves. Data on suicide linked to specific events in Zimbabwe (or anywhere, for that matter) is poorly documented. However, between 2006 and 2008, the World Health Organization shared suicide statistics for Africa, and Zimbabwe had one of the highest rates on the continent. Ultimately, even though I didn't have the language for it at the time, what I wanted to do was save lives and break cycles. After Erica's death, I slowly recognized that a dramatic intervention needed to take place at the community level, not just the individual one. An intervention is an action that public health professionals take on behalf of individuals, families, and communities to measurably improve health. We had to find a way of taking evidence-based mental healthcare from the hospital right into the community, so it could be within walking distance for all. I had no idea how it would unfold, but I was ready for the challenge ahead of me. I wanted to do whatever I could to make sure that as many people as possible would be spared the same fate as Erica.

In early 2006, the Harare city health department was happy to support an initiative to heal the community trauma resulting from Murambatsvina. They were keen to save face because they were aligned to the ruling party responsible for the cleanup, and I happened to be in the right place at the right time. I wanted to do something about Erica's suicide, although her death had nothing to do with Murambatsvina. Rather, my desire to help was part of a private internal battle, and I saw my participation in a citywide initiative to be an atonement of sorts. Conveniently, at the time, I was the only psychiatrist in Zimbabwe who worked in the public health sector. At a presentation on the psychological effects of Murambatsvina on communities across the country, I committed to coming up with a solution that would be simple and cost-effective, though I was clueless as to what it might be.

At first, the director of city health services made it clear to me that I would not be receiving any funding to support my initiative, as the department had no budget for a community mental health initiative. He was, however, sympathetic and recognized that too many people had been affected by the atrocities of the past several months. Unfortunately, the city health department was already overwhelmed with many other civic issues, particularly with respect to HIV/AIDS, maternal and child health, tuberculosis, and the kinds of conditions and infectious diseases that are common in low-income settings with overcrowding and little infrastructure. Still, he acknowledged the need to do something and was willing to give my work a needed platform.

Despite the absence of material or financial resources, I was appreciative. Perhaps the initiative would gain steam if more people learned about it, but that would also mean I'd have to come up with a strong enough idea for an intervention.

Apart from some initial monetary support from a local NGO, the first few years of running this initiative were funded directly out of my government salary from the work I was still doing at the hospital during my shifts every Thursday. I felt I owed that much to Erica. In a country where most young people had left for greener pastures — primarily South Africa, the United Kingdom, and Australia — the elderly were the most likely target for my experimental intervention. This was the beginning of what would eventually come to be called the Friendship Bench.

My original idea was that, in the absence of funding, I could train a handful of nurses in the basics of cognitive behavioral therapy (CBT) so that they'd be able to provide an evidence-based mental health intervention in a primary care setting. However, after it was decided that I would start the initiative in Mbare, one of the most densely populated suburbs and the most affected community in Harare, I learned that I couldn't include the trained staff of nurses and doctors working within this community, as they were already overwhelmed with other projects.

I didn't despair for long. I was informed that a group of fourteen grandmothers had volunteered their time around interventions focused on health education and awareness across Mbare. The City of Harare worked with these grandmothers from time to time to promote adherence to HIV medication; the women were pillars in their communities, and people were likely to pay their words heed. I jotted down their contact information and took time to visit each of them. Having witnessed the destruction that had impacted their communities in the past several months (and, indeed, long before), they were eager to help. Eventually, we were all able to meet at the local clinic, which was where we began discussing in earnest how this entire program could unfold.

Ours was an extremely informal arrangement without any bureaucratic hoops to jump through. In fact, none of the grandmothers seemed to be interested in a formal agreement at all — they didn't want any part in that. They simply believed that doing the work was good for them. It gave them a sense of meaning, purpose, and belonging in their communities. As custodians of their local culture, they felt responsible for creating community cohesion by giving back to the people around them.

I was immediately struck by the wisdom of the fourteen grandmothers. Altogether, if you were to add up their ages, they were proprietors of a collective treasury of more than a thousand years' worth of experience. I quickly learned from them that mental health was simply an entry point into story-telling — a timeless communal tool that had been forgotten by many Zimbabweans but that had the potential to trans-form individuals, families, and communities who had borne the brunt of the damage. These grandmothers showed me that there were many ways of unpacking CBT. When we started, it did not occur to me that for our work to succeed we had to be authentically immersed in the local culture. We had to create an indigenous CBT approach that would not alienate us from the community. Traditional CBT is based on the link between our thoughts, feelings, and behavior — how they are all interconnected and influence our outlook on life — with a particular focus on bringing our distorted thoughts more in line with reality.

The grandmothers, through decades of lived experience, had developed an internal compass, a culturally rooted sys-tem to navigate through the emotional and psychological issues presented to them — a higher level of psychological consciousness, if you like. They possessed an ability to intu-itively see the link between feelings, thoughts, moods, and behavior and to apply this intuitive ability in their problem-solving therapy. They also understood that a shift would come through breaking the cycle of negative thoughts and feelings at the behavior level by scheduling activities, such as garden-ing or going to the local community clubs, that would lead to positive, rewarding behavior. While they were never trained to be professional CBT therapists, they inherently grasped the fundamental building blocks of CBT, that link between positive activity and improved mental well-being.

Of course, by their nature, grandmothers are firm in their hard-earned knowledge and have strong convictions that can make them stubborn — and at times difficult to work with.

The most difficult of the fourteen grandmothers by far was Grandmother Jack, a headstrong and combative eighty-two-year-old who wore her signature red beret everywhere. She'd lived in Mbare all her life and had many insights to share. Although I initially found some of her ways of communicating these insights to be irksome and even hostile, she would prove to be a powerful thought leader who had the tenacity of a revolutionary thinker. In some ways, she would be my greatest teacher as I transitioned from hospital-based to community-based mental healthcare.

Psychiatry, like any other science, is anchored in empirical observation, using proven tools that are routinely accepted in the trade. The problem, according to the grandmothers, was one that many postcolonial scholars and other contemporary thinkers are familiar with: What exactly was "empirical" observation, and who was defining it?

Initially, during one of their first trainings in basic problem-solving therapy, I suggested finding a clinic in which to offer the intervention to community members. Grandmother Jack challenged me with fiery eyes: "With everything demolished here, why would you think of delivering therapy in some building?" Shaking her head, she went on: "You're thinking too much like a doctor when you say we should find an empty office or room in the clinic. Our people have always used the outdoors to share stories and resolve conflict."

I knew she was right. In many African and low-income countries, ancestral spirits are connected to the land; nature was the perfect backdrop for the kind of work that most Western-trained physicians like myself would certainly have conducted in a more "clinical" setting. It was also the most pragmatic, considering the lack of easy access to "proper" facilities. In fact, Grandmother Jack's challenge to me became a blessing in disguise, because it turned out that the authorities never actually intended to provide us with any working space within the city's clinic buildings.

Still, I struggled. It was obvious to the grandmothers I was using my highly clinical approach to try to create something within the community, and I encountered resistance at every step. For example, I was accustomed to using jargon from the ICD-10 (the tenth revision of the *International Classification of Diseases and Related Health Problems*) and the DSM-4 (the fourth edition of the *Diagnostic and Statistical Manual of Mental Disorders*) to label and diagnose my patients, but the grandmothers were not interested in this at all. In fact, they thought these diagnostic tools were a total waste of time. They preferred that our intervention provide a platform for encouraging people to tell their stories and to experience the catharsis of being truly heard and held. It took me a while to recognize that although the aim of our intervention was to help people who were struggling with depression and other common mental disorders, there were many creative ways to go about fulfilling this purpose. This isn't a new idea. For example, the interdisciplinary field of narrative medicine uses skills like storytelling, empathy, and listening to provide transformative spaces to those who both seek and offer healthcare.

What the grandmothers helped me to see, and what I eventually began to appreciate, was that these skills had existed within the cultures of Zimbabwe and many other African countries since time immemorial. Oral storytelling has always been an important aspect of our spiritual and secular lives. To this day, I remember sitting with my own grandmother around a fire, listening with rapt attention as she told a story — usually a fable about animals engaged in different activities that eventually culminated in a fundamental lesson about the power of community.

I came to see that the focus on the use of "developed" Western medical frameworks had removed us from the therapeutic benefits of storytelling that were already rooted within our ancestral traditions.

Moreover, as a practitioner of Western medicine, I came to see that I myself was guilty of devaluing our cultural methods — I had never considered that storytelling could be a way of moving beyond treating symptoms and getting to root causes. In fact, in a Western medical setting, storytelling was discouraged. Of course, if you were a medical anthropologist, you understood the importance of narratives in getting to the bottom of a pathology, but even this approach to storytelling was mechanical and structured — a means to an end, more than anything.

Another thing that struck me about the grandmothers as I got to know them was that they weren't interested in storytelling as a modality to "fix" or "cure" anything. They were simply invested in being present for the person to whom they were speaking, expressing empathy, and allowing the other to feel acknowledged.

And so it went: through our spirited meetings, many of which were not without disagreement, the grandmothers would help me to fully feel and realize the transformative power of a good story.

It took about three months before Grandmother Jack's astute observations started to make sense to me. It was at this point that the idea of trained grandmothers providing therapy in their communities — and from wooden park benches rather than fusty rooms inside a clinic — emerged.

Together, we iterated on the first pilot of the Friendship Bench — which actually comprised five benches altogether, sitting outside of three clinics in Mbare. Each of the grandmothers was given a set of shifts, enabling them to attend to anyone who wanted to come, sit down, and talk about their problems. True to form, the grandmothers fought me on my initial name for the initiative: I wanted to call it the Mental Health Bench. The grandmothers insisted that Friendship Bench was a nonstigmatizing name that people would resonate with; it was welcoming and approachable, and it would ensure that people actually came back! I grudgingly agreed and quickly came to see the wisdom behind their suggestion (or, rather, their demand!).

Aside from Grandmother Jack, Grandmother Hwiza was an imperative part of the plan and a testament to the endurance of the women who would be at the forefront of the intervention. *Hwiza* means "grasshopper" in the Shona language.

Granny Grasshopper had been tortured during the liberation war by Rhodesian Prime Minister Ian Smith's police force for harboring so-called terrorists; according to her (and to so many others, including my own grandmother), the "terrorists" were actually freedom fighters.

Grandmother Hwiza informed us that the freedom fighters chose her house because of her son, who had been discreetly communicating with them. "They had come in from Tete Province in Mozambique," where the base for the freedom fighters was situated. "There were originally eight of them but only four stayed at my house," she said, lowering her voice, suddenly hypervigilant, as if she feared someone might overhear.

The four had stayed in her house for almost a week as they planned their attack. Her job was to feed them and keep the neighborhood unsuspecting. A few days later, the only fuel-storage depot with a capacity of more than 100,000 liters of fuel was blown up in Salisbury (now Harare), resulting in a massive fuel shortage that marked the beginning of the end of the Ian Smith government on that fateful day: December 11, 1978.

The incident also changed Grandmother Hwiza's life, particularly after she was tortured for her participation.

"Sometimes you stay up all night," she said softly during one of the group meetings with the other grandmothers, "and sleeping makes you relive the experience over and over again as you dream." But immediately after these words, she smiled and broke into song and dance, as if to disrupt the negative energy and channel it in a different direction. The others simultaneously joined in, each one instinctively knowing where to place her voice in the soothing chorus.

"In times of trouble, singing, dancing, and praying to-gether can be better therapy than seeing a psychiatrist," Grandmother Hwiza said with affectionate mockery as she pointed at me while continuing to move to the rhythm. She had lost all her front teeth from the physical abuse inflicted on her while she was in custody, but they hadn't managed to beat the light and life out of her. Whenever I saw her, I was greeted by her magnanimous grin, which filled our little corner with warmth and affection every time she spoke.

Grandmother Chinhoyi was another memorable grand-mother; she refused to work with material that was not writ-ten in the local Shona language, although she was fluent in English. Her argument was that "emotional problems are best said in your own language." Grandmother Chinhoyi was also secretly referred to as "the peanut butter machine lady" by her peers after she took ownership of a peanut butter machine that had been donated to the group. Her argument: she was the only one who knew how to use it!

I could readily see, without having to get into the minu-tiae of these women's stories and backgrounds, that they were spirited and resilient. Within their communities, they'd been witness to a number of festering traumas: a high prevalence of HIV/AIDS, violence against women, and, now, the displace-ment and stress that were the end result of Murambatsvina.

They all seemed to proclaim that when you've lived this long and seen this much, you don't get bent out of shape by difficult experiences or unfavorable circumstances as much as you otherwise would. They enjoyed strong relationships with the people in their community; because of this, and despite the poverty they'd all faced to some extent, they were assured that through every hardship and trauma, many people — even those with few resources beyond their kindness and hard-earned life experience — had their back.

I quickly realized that every single one of my collaborators felt the responsibility necessary to create a collective sense of belonging. And that was the key: although it is normally assumed that the elders in a community need assistance, these grandmothers weren't just seeking support — they understood that they were also the ones offering it.

I was quickly coming to appreciate that my Western model of care, which had not considered the value of local knowledge and wisdom, was insufficient for dealing with the many problems that were facing the communities I sought to help. With a communal approach such as that which the grandmothers could offer, there would be a safe space for grief to land and be expressed.

The idea of the Friendship Bench was now more than just an idea: it was something we were ready to tailor to the community.

While the grandmothers and I certainly didn't agree on everything, at least at first, we did come to an agreement that the screening tool I'd offered for common mental disorders, the Shona Symptom Questionnaire (SSQ-14), was a pertinent guide that could help them establish a sense of the severity of symptoms induced by social determinants — in other words, the severity of the clients' mental health struggle. The SSQ-14 was a set of fourteen questions that inquired how a person had been feeling in the past seven days within such areas of their lives as sleep, mood, suicidal thoughts, hallucinations, motivation, and physical symptoms, among others. At the start of the project, clinic nurses from various facilities administered the questionnaire, which led to countless referrals to the Friendship Bench. Over time, we ended up getting self-referrals via word of mouth, and as the intervention became more popular, the grandmothers themselves offered the SSQ-14 to patients who came to them.

However, the grandmothers strongly felt that whatever issue a client might bring to them did not necessarily have to be attached to a clinical condition. Grandmother Jack was adamant that depression was a Western concept that didn't resonate with her community. "You can't use those terms here! They won't mean anything to people needing emotional support," she insisted.

One of the common symptoms of depression is "over-thinking," a term commonly referred to as *kufungisisa* in Shona. While the grandmothers recognized that it often accompanied stressful situations, they didn't see it as the primary symptom of an illness at all. Rather, it was a natural response to a wide range of social, family, political, and economic challenges that people were facing — something I had also come to think about more deeply in the wake of Murambatsvina, as well as the loss of Erica.

"The problem itself is the thing that causes the kufungisisa," Grandmother Jack explained. So focusing on the symptoms was meaningless when a person was depressed because they were HIV positive and couldn't get the support they needed to live well with HIV, or they were in an abusive relationship and the community was just watching from a distance. Collective community response, she said, "is what will help most of the kufungisisa that people are facing. This is where *kuvhura pfungwa* [opening the mind] becomes important."

Grandmother Kusi, who was always immaculately dressed no matter what the occasion, chimed in: "Yes! See, the average person coming to the bench does not want treatment for depression. They want treatment for their problems with money and people, and that is why it is better to offer them kuvhura pfungwa. Opening the mind is what leads to seeing clearly and realizing that they can do something about their unhappiness."

The term *kuvhura pfungwa* had first been used in our meetings when Grandmother Jack, in her typically candid fashion, pointed out my failure to see the big picture. "We all need to open our minds," she had said, smiling, "for only by opening our minds can we see the resources that are in each person, family, and community."

Later on, together with the other grandmothers, she would consistently talk about kuvhura pfungwa to describe the first step of therapy that was necessary to create space for people to share their stories on the Friendship Bench.

"So what drives kuvhura pfungwa?" I asked the grandmothers one morning as we sat in the shed outside the clinic where we were now convening our regular meetings.

"Empathy that's said out loud, not just felt," responded Grandmother Jack.

"Making people feel respected and understood, regardless of their money or status or the problems they bring to the bench," added Grandmother Kusi.

"The most difficult thing to do when talking to a person is noticing how we are judging them inside," said Grandmother Hwiza. "And then, just being there and sending them empathy without judging them. We all struggle with this as humans, but ultimately, that is the highest level of kuvhura pfungwa. With all our imperfections, this is what we should strive for."

"You know, Doctor, we all have that quick tendency to judge. I guess it's our way of being seen to be in the right," Grandmother Jack went on, "but I think with age, you learn to judge less. We hear about all sorts of dirt happening in the community, and we become that ear that everyone needs."

I nodded as I took in the grandmothers' words. "But what is it that makes you become less judgmental with age?"

"Well, when you're old and ready to move on to the next world, you have seen so much and done so much that very little can shock you!" said Grandmother Jack.

"People worry more about things that haven't actually happened," said Grandmother Chizhande, who had a coarse voice but often gentle words to offer. "It's the fear of the unknown that kills us most of the time."

"And also, when you are old, everybody thinks you know everything," Grandmother Jack added, "but the truth is, there is still a lot we don't know — we're just more likely not to panic in the face of disaster!"

"That is *exactly* what a person is looking for when they come to the Friendship Bench." Grandmother Kusi sounded excited. "Sometimes, even when we have no idea what needs to happen, just listening makes a big difference, especially for people who are lonely."

I was beginning to understand why the grandmothers felt

that healing could begin only when a client was able to share their story. And it was impossible to share an emotional story with someone who didn't express empathy, who didn't make the person in need feel, as Grandmother Kusi had said, respected and understood. I began to wonder whether or not I had shared my support with Erica and others to the best of my ability, especially given that I'd always been trained to keep interactions with patients clean and simple — just the facts, ma'am.

"It's also about the power of the human voice. You need to understand how to use it as a tool," said Grandmother Jack. "The voice can be medicine."

As I listened to them talk, I learned that the grandmothers believed the way one spoke to another person had a greater impact than structured therapy — and this included the timbre of the voice, the words used, the body language displayed, and, of course, the eye contact made. These were tools innate to every human being, but a lot of people had lost the ability to use them, often because of trauma and the destruction of supportive communities of people.

"How does the training you received help? And does it help at all?" I inquired. I myself had offered their initial training, along with two clinical psychologists.

"The training and the tools help to give structure," Grandmother Hwiza replied, "especially that screening tool! Those fourteen questions help me to see how severe a situation is. But you still want to focus on the story and on listening."

"The other thing I think is important from the training is the idea of the summary," added Grandmother Kusi, referring to the practice of listening to a client's story and then summarizing what they said back to them. "That can really help them to feel heard and even give them a new understanding." She sighed. "People facing challenges have not often had the opportunity to sit and tell their story to a person who is genuinely interested in helping them."

As I sat in the presence of the grandmothers, I wondered if I had done enough. Grandmother Jack's gaze at me was piercing but kind, as if she could feel the guilt I still carried about Erica. "If the story is real and true empathy is conveyed," she said, "that's where the healing actually starts."

There was a rich and detailed story — of suffering, hope, and resilience — connected to every single grandmother who sat with me around the circle as we discussed the mental health intervention we would be offering. Grandmother Makokoba, commonly referred to as Mako by her peers, suffered from chronic arthritis. Each week, during our debriefing sessions, she would indicate the part of her body that was in pain before sharing her experiences on the bench. I could tell from her gnarled fingers and the way she sometimes labored through our conversations that her pain was no small thing. However, the stories that she told were transmitted from every part of her being, especially through her raucous laugh, which would resonate through each of our sessions.

"You won't believe what happened just yesterday," she started one day as she proudly adjusted the Friendship Bench

T-shirt that she wore. It acted as an advertisement for the service we wished to provide to the people of the community. "This young man — he's twenty-four. He lost his house during Murambatsvina, like most people. He used to be self-employed, selling solar lights, but lost all his products and his cash when his house was demolished. Now, he has been selling his body to survive."

"Like a woman?" Grandmother Hwiza asked. Although male prostitution was not unheard of in Zimbabwe and had been on the rise because of the country's collapsed economy, it still came as a bit of a surprise to the grandmothers.

"Yes," Grandmother Mako replied. "But now, listen. He was found having sex with that businessman who owns the big grinding mill at the corner!"

A chorus of "Mai wheee!" came from the other thirteen grannies before Grandmother Jack nonchalantly added, "Well, we've always known that particular businessman does men. So what's the deal?"

Mako lowered her voice. "It was the businessman's *wife* who caught them! They were at it behind the grinding mill."

There was silence followed by muttering as the women pondered this juicy piece of community gossip.

"So tell me, what is worse?" asked Grandmother Kusi with a twitch of mischief. "To find your man with a woman or with a man?"

Grandmother Jack smirked and shrugged. "It's all sex, isn't it? Only difference is that with one form, no one will get pregnant!" She looked at Grandmother Kusi, her eyes full of curiosity. "What did he want?"

"He was referred by the clinic nurse because he had an

SSQ of ten," Grandmother Kusi replied. Now, I was curious, too. Such a high score on the questionnaire meant he was clearly in need of help. "He wanted to talk. He lost his home a month ago, and for the past three weeks, he was miserable. The businessman had abandoned him!"

"What did you decide after hearing his story?" Grandmother Jack pressed on.

"I didn't decide anything. He said he wanted to speak to men who sleep with other men, so I referred him to GALZ."

GALZ is an organization that serves the needs of the lesbian, gay, bisexual, transgender, and intersex community in Zimbabwe. Established in 1990 in Harare, it was meant to counter many of the still pervasive prejudices that gay and trans people might encounter in traditional communities. During the grandmothers' training, we'd talked about the importance of referrals to other organizations and collectives that might be better equipped than us to address a client's specific situation.

"It's strange that a person can be into men and not even know about GALZ," Grandmother Mako quipped.

"Knowledge is power." Grandmother Jack smiled.

"Did he go?" I asked, eager to learn how this particular story ended.

"Yes, he did! He sent me a message saying he had been and he would come back to talk to me in two days' time. He sounded grateful." Grandmother Mako looked proud.

"These outdoor sex escapades have increased after Murambatsvina," Grandmother Chizhande observed. She was not the most outspoken of the grandmothers, but she was the one who would eventually emphasize the importance of interacting with clients beyond the Friendship Bench alone; she saw value in going into their homes and providing groups that would offer psychosocial support and a sense of deep belonging. "Now, you see people having sex along the Mukuvisi River," she went on. "With all the homes destroyed, you see condoms thrown everywhere by the river because they can't go do it in private."

"At least they're using condoms," Grandmother Jack pointed out, finding a rare silver lining in a dismal situation. The prevalence of HIV in people between fifteen and forty-nine years of age in Zimbabwe was 15 percent. All of the grandmothers had tended to family members dying of HIV/AIDS.

"The Mukuvisi River area stinks. I just don't get how people can be intimate at a place like that," said Grandmother Mako, sadly shaking her head.

"Well, when your whole body is focused on the genitals, your ability to distinguish between good and bad smell is impaired," joked Grandmother Jack.

"And when you hang around a smelly place long enough, the smell starts to feel like home!" exclaimed Grandmother Kusi.

"A bit like your own fart," added Grandmother Mako, sending all the grandmothers into a raucous fit of laughter.

"I want to share my debrief, too." Grandmother Chizhande interrupted the jovial mood. "This woman was referred to me by the clinic nurse. One day she'd come home and found some weird concoction of herbs tied around the foot of the bed. From the minute she saw this, she started having these attacks, where her heart would beat fast and she would feel terrified — she thought she was going to die. She said she had been bewitched."

I nodded, urging her to continue. I understood that superstitions about "black magic" abounded in the community, and I knew that sensitivity and discretion around such topics were paramount.

"I gave her the SSQ, and it was eleven points. She answered yes to the suicidal question," Chizhande said. "When I told her that her SSQ score was high and she definitely had issues with kufungisisa, she broke down crying. We decided to pray." While this wouldn't be advisable in a clinical setting, most patients seemed to appreciate the grandmothers' suggestion to pray, which often felt like a loving nudge in the direction of an empowering solution.

"So I held her hand, and we prayed together. Then she opened up more and told me a traditional healer had advised her to go to her ancestral home and pour some opaque beer [a traditional brew made from malted sorghum] on her mother's grave. Alas, she didn't have the money to get on a bus. We brainstormed on how to get her home, because this was the issue she wanted to deal with. She decided to sell one of her pairs of shoes at the flea market."

"Did it work?"

"She managed to raise the six dollars for the bus to her village. She left yesterday."

Grandmother Chizhande's story immediately made me think of Erica and her mother. I felt a sense of relief that Chizhande's patient had found a way to collect the money she needed.

"And when will you follow up with her?" inquired Grandmother Jack.

"I should know in another few days, but she was quite relieved to have the money."

As the grandmothers continued to debrief, I reflected that one thing was certain. While each of them had their own unique style, and their responses varied depending on what the person sitting next to them needed, they were empowering the people in their midst by allowing them to feel heard, seen, and affirmed.

Many who came in search of counsel and connection were facing a confluence of issues, so people often returned to the Friendship Bench over and over again. "This idea of having a nice little list of problems is very academic, but in real life, it never works like that," Grandmother Komai said during one of our meetings.

Grandmother Komai was tall, dark, and elegant. She spoke softly, and unlike the opinionated and passionate Grandmother Jack, she often preferred to listen and contributed only when she had substantial news to share. "Let me tell you, Doctor. Just last week, this young man was referred to the bench by the nurse from the clinic across the road. He was a victim of domestic violence."

The other grandmothers snickered at the notion of a man being beaten up by his wife. I reminded myself that they weren't trained clinicians and in some ways had bought into the prejudices of the larger community, despite their general empathy and efficacy.

Grandmother Komai looked sternly at her peers. "This is serious! Stop laughing! This young man has become a laughingstock at work and the local pub. It's also known that his wife has a boyfriend. He started taking a lot of cannabis to try to forget about his wife's mischief, as he puts it. Then he was fired at work for performing poorly, and now the wife is telling him to go to the village, to move out of the house, because he is a burden."

The grandmothers were silent now, sobered by Grandmother Komai's story. She paused, as if to absorb the gravity of the problem. "He was referred to me by the clinic nurse because he was a red flag, according to the SSQ. He responded yes to the question about being suicidal."

Grandmother Jack's eyes widened. "So he wants to kill himself because his wife has a side man? Imagine how many women would kill themselves in Mbare if they reacted like him at the side chicks all their men have!"

"Zvakaoma se munamato," Grandmother Hwiza said — a Shona saying that translates to, "It's as difficult as praying." Commonly espoused by the grandmothers when they were huddled in discussion or conversing with me, it suggested the challenge or impossibility of a situation.

"How did you handle this one?" I asked.

"I told him, 'I'm here for you — you can share your story.' He started narrating his childhood, which was also quite abusive, and then he broke down and cried. I told him it was OK to cry."

"Kuvhura pfungwa right there!" exclaimed Grandmother Chinhoyi, impressed by Grandmother Komai's compassionate and gentle response — especially given the fact that many Zimbabwean men might have felt emasculated by such a suggestion. However, the grandmothers knew something that many women who have watched over generations of family members understand very well: it's healthy and safe to cry. In fact, it often relieves us of the stress and pain that come from restraining our feelings and pretending they don't exist.

"Yes," responded Grandmother Komai. "After he cried and seemed content, he shared his full story. Then I asked him to choose one problem he wanted to start working on."

"And?" asked Grandmother Jack impatiently.

"This is the part where I think the training we received falls short." Grandmother Komai looked directly at me.

"Tell me more," I encouraged her.

"When a person shows up with numerous problems and all of them seem quite serious…" Her voice trailed off.

"Can you give me an example?" I asked.

"Well, you know, like someone is HIV positive, they are unemployed, they are in an abusive relationship, they have a teenage daughter who is pregnant — you know — all these problems and more! When you have such a cocktail of problems and you ask a person which problem they would like to work on first, they sometimes panic from sheer helplessness. That's when you get into the here-there, here-there exchange."

"What do you mean?"

"Kunge ka bhora kanenge kachiti uko, apo, uko, kwese kwese," Grandmother Komai exclaimed. This roughly translates to, "Like a ball all over the place, like Ping-Pong."

"Ping-Pong? I don't understand."

"Let me explain," Grandmother Kusi offered. "So you

know when the client says, 'I don't know which problem to focus on, all of them are important,' and we say we need to start with one, and the client says, 'Can you choose for me?' and I say, 'I can't possibly put myself in your shoes, no matter how hard I try, so you have to decide which one you want to start working on'?" She imitated the movement of a ball back and forth with her hands.

"And that can go on for a long while," added Grandmother Komai. "It's a pattern. We've seen it in a lot of the clients. It's like they're carrying many sacks of heavy stuff and they feel they can't put any of them down. So the trick is to help them to let go." She opened her arms and breathed deeply, as if she were releasing a burden.

"The process of getting them to let go of all but one is part of kuvhura pfungwa," explained Grandmother Hwiza. "This is how you help them to see there is another way to deal with their problems."

"But sometimes, they resist," said Grandmother Kusi. "And sometimes, you just sit and listen to them talk and talk about why they can't let go of any of their problems. You just listen, until suddenly" — she clasped her hands together in an energetic gesture — "they get it and they say, 'I will start with *this* problem!'"

After a thoughtful pause, Grandmother Jack offered, "In a way, this therapy is not so much problem-solving but really helping people to let go. Unless you can let go, you can't solve the problems, so accepting the need to let go comes first — and that is kuvhura pfungwa."

I nodded. "Letting go makes a lot of sense," I said. "But what would you say is the main thing that people have to let go of, that brings them to the Friendship Bench in the first place? The challenge they most struggle to release?"

"Poverty," replied Grandmother Kusi. This was followed by the traditional "Hongu" ("Oh yes") of agreement from the others. "People here are poor, but when you also have poverty of thought, then you are truly screwed," she added.

"How do you deal with poverty? I mean, how do you use the skills you were taught, together with your collective knowledge and wisdom, to address poverty?" I realized I'd never delved so deeply into this topic, not even with the clinicians I knew.

"Kutambura chiremba kuri mupfungwa," said Grandmother Jack — "Poverty is in the mind."

"The worst is when people come to the bench and define themselves through the lens of poverty," Grandmother Kusi said with a sigh, "especially these young people. They are so lost."

"But *why* are they lost?" I wanted to understand something the grandmothers seemed to have direct, lived experience with but that still felt elusive to me.

Grandmother Hwiza cleared her throat. "From what I've seen, they don't have anchors in the community." This elicited another enthusiastic "Hongu" from the group. "They want to belong; they want to have meaning and purpose. And when they can't find that, they turn to what is easily available — the things that help to numb the mind." I knew what she meant by this. In general, these "things" encompassed a range of substances, from alcohol to codeine to cannabis to crystal meth. There was a serious substance abuse problem in Zimbabwe that had increased in the past few years. I had seen the numbers shift dramatically, and I understood that Muram-batsvina probably had something to do with it.

"This is why kuvhura pfungwa is important — because when your mind is open, you see clearly and you can focus on one thing at a time," Grandmother Hwiza concluded.

It made absolute sense. As a psychiatrist, I understood the importance and power of asking a client to slow down and breathe, so as to halt a cascade of catastrophic thoughts and allow them to focus on what was immediate and present. I was moved by the grandmothers' understanding of this process and their ability to be with someone under duress, accompanying them with such presence and compassion.

Grandmother Jack piped up. "The three most relevant steps that help us to address these issues are kuvhura pfungwa [opening the mind], *kusimudzira* [to uplift], and *kusimbisa* [to strengthen]. These are the three most important pillars of the therapy we provide on the bench!"

Grandmother Kusi nodded. "And when we use these terms, it removes the stigma that is associated with going to, say, a psychiatrist like you," she added, gracing me with a playful smile. "These people feel a lot more comfortable sitting on a wooden bench and talking about their life challenges with a grandmother, using language they can identify with."

I thought about how I'd initially been skeptical of the grandmothers' capacity to reserve their judgments against LGBTQ people or sex workers — people who were already marginalized by their communities because of traditional attitudes or simple ignorance. But I understood that even when the grandmothers laughed or gossiped, they took their responsibility as stewards of their community's mental health very seriously. I also came to realize that many of the concerns I'd had were not quite as applicable to the context of a community in Zimbabwe as I'd initially believed. Over and over again, the grandmothers would insist that terms like *LGBTQ* and *sex workers* were merely Western labels for identities that had existed in Africa since time immemorial.

The depth of their lived experience was profound. I had little doubt that many of them had faced the same issues they were counseling others to move through: domestic violence, poverty, disease, sexual shaming, and the list went on. I continued to be astonished by the way they could hold difficult experiences with reverence, which was perhaps how they had been able to make the Friendship Bench such an essential anchor in the community.

At the same time that they held all manner of deep tragedy with compassion, they were not bereft of levity. I was familiar with the concept of compassion fatigue, the phenomenon of secondhand stress and trauma that results from helping others who are going through difficult situations; it's something that many mental health workers struggle with. But I marveled at the effortless way in which the grandmothers could create a safe space for their clients' sharing without being negatively affected or letting them take a toll on their own well-being. It wasn't unusual for them to suddenly get up and break into song and dance when they debriefed together or when they were discussing difficult cases with me. This custom came from traditional African funerals and other ritualized events. It provided a cathartic release of any residual emotions that might be lingering — a very different approach from the Western model of sitting in a hushed room and talking matter-of-factly about difficult emotions.

And, as the grandmothers would constantly and gently remind me, "At our age, we've seen everything! Not only have we seen everything — we've done everything." This would invariably be followed by a fit of cackles and giggles, which would in turn make me smile and soften, feeling reassured that I was in the right place with just the right people to provide the help their community so desperately needed.

Intuitively, over a six-month period, the fourteen grandmothers created their own mental health lexicon. It would be a while, however, before it was formally integrated into the program — especially because I worried my work wouldn't be accepted by the global mental health community if I strayed from using only the prescribed frameworks for interventions. But whatever they were doing, it was working. In just a few months of the Friendship Bench being available to the community, they had served more than three thousand Mbare residents.

I spent most of my days in Mbare interacting with the grandmothers. During the formative years of the Friendship Bench, I was particularly fortunate to work with Petra Mesu and Lazarus Kajawu, two clinical psychologists who were instrumental in encouraging me to carry on with the grandmothers after the modest funding we received from a local NGO was terminated.

I recall Petra telling me, "If you don't continue, all the progress you've made will collapse. I don't know how you're going to keep doing it, but you have to — and you're the only one who can."

Petra had played a leading role in putting together our first protocol for problem-solving therapy, which was what the grandmothers would go on to adapt by using more appropriate, culturally aligned idioms of distress.

An idiom of distress is a culturally bound statement that speaks to the presence of mental fatigue or stress, using the vernacular and lingo of a specific group of people. This is extremely important, as a clinician who's more versed in the terms of the dominant culture might completely miss symptoms of depression or anxiety if they're depending primarily on the DSM for the language that fits what they might be looking for. It's not unusual across many African cultures for people to resort to colorful metaphors to describe their experiences. The grandmothers understood that someone who came to the Friendship Bench might not speak directly about depression, but statements like "I have a painful heart" or "My spirits have abandoned me" might suggest that depression was present.

My Thursdays remained dedicated to my work at the hospital, where I continued to run an outpatient clinic and manage patients who had been admitted that Monday. But each week spent with the grandmothers iterating on how best to reach the people in the greatest need gradually led me to a powerful and humbling realization: the mental health problems of most of the people coming to my outpatient clinic could be managed in their communities, without a psychiatrist getting involved at all. And perhaps, in the process, they might find themselves in the loving and capable hands of a grandmother who would empower them to recognize that solutions, even if they felt out of reach, were in fact available to them.

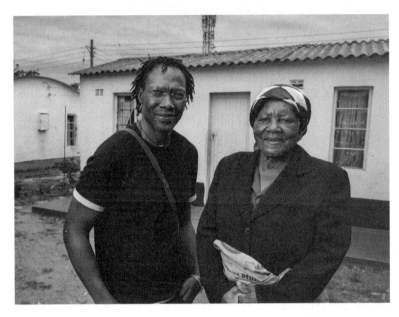

Visiting Grandmother Hwiza at her house in Mbare in 2019. She had lived in this house since 1951. It was from here that she planned the attack on the fuel-storage depot in 1978.

Chapter Four

Pineapples and Voodoo

Nearly a year after the inception of the Friendship Bench, my work with the grandmothers was going well, and I could feel it beginning to shift my experience of myself. I had a newfound sense of purpose, peace, and possibility. Although I was working behind the scenes with the Friendship Bench, providing training and feedback to the grandmothers during our debriefing sessions every week, I was starting to feel the inklings of a new movement that could easily stretch beyond Mbare and positively impact other people in Zimbabwe, perhaps even elsewhere in the world. Maybe we'd be able to share a therapy that had at its core the notion of kuvhura pfungwa — that opening of the mind that came through the power of having one's story heard and held with compassion and acceptance, leading to a change in a client's perspective.

I could feel my initial reservations melt away and, with them, some of the professionalism that at times held me back from the engaged empathy that the grandmothers were teaching me. As I spent more time with them, listening to them share stories about clients who came to them with problems but left with a sense of empowerment, slowly but surely my own perspectives were evolving. New dimensions were starting to open up in my approach to the therapeutic model; I didn't feel so constrained to the protocols I'd learned in medical school, protocols that I'd been indoctrinated to believe were the only legitimate ones. And I was getting in touch with my vulnerability, which helped me to relax a little and let down my guard with the grandmothers.

But there was still something that didn't release its grip on my heart: my regret for not having acted sooner to prevent Erica's death.

Although I dealt with other difficult stories in my work as a psychiatrist, Erica's death continued to touch me deeply, mostly because she and her family knew she needed help, but economic hardship had prevented her from getting it. I needed an escape from the tragic reality that Erica was no longer with us. Most of all, I needed a way to forget my failure. My work with the fourteen grandmothers from Mbare was a good distraction, a worthy one — but I still had to come to the hospital every Thursday to run my clinic. The rawness of the loss came to the surface every time I made my rounds. On some level, I saw it as the punishment I would endure for the rest of my professional career. I only hoped that with the work I was doing with the grandmothers, the pain of Erica's loss would gradually be appeased.

Something that would both reopen that wound and help me begin to heal it occurred during those early stages of the

Friendship Bench. Erica's mother, Sekai, paid me an unexpected visit on a Thursday morning at Harare Central Hospital. She patiently waited until after the clinic was over; when the last outpatient walked out, she asked to speak with me.

Sekai sat in the corner where she'd normally sat when she'd accompanied Erica to our sessions. She looked frail and lifeless. I could see in her face that within the past few months, she had become a changed woman. So much had occurred — so much that no mother should ever have to face.

A brief silence transpired, but it felt like hours. We gazed at each other. I didn't know what to say. Words felt so trivial compared to the understanding that passed between us in those few moments.

She looked at me the way a mother looks at her helpless child. With a soft smile, she said, "I have brought you a pineapple!"

My eyes welled with tears. I was moved that in the midst of her grief, she'd thought to give me this one indulgence. "I'm sorry," I managed to say, my voice cracking.

She didn't have to respond; the wrinkles in her face shifted her expression. She seemed to have aged in such a short period of time. Tears trickled down her cheeks as she silently wept. I reached out to hold her hand, knowing that it wasn't enough. Instinctively, both of us stood, and I held her close as she broke down. Her tiny body smelled of smoke from a traditional African kitchen. I continued to hold her as I looked at the pineapple she had placed on my desk. By now, both of us were openly sobbing.

It was a strange experience. I felt very exposed, very vulnerable — and I somehow knew this was exactly what I needed in order to break through the fragile veneer of my professionalism. Perhaps I had needed it ever since learning about Erica's death, but I couldn't have asked for such a thing months ago. I had tried to maintain the facade of professionalism to the best of my ability, perhaps to my own detriment. As Sekai and I stood there, a wave of relief washed over me. I could feel that she didn't blame me for her daughter's death. The fact that she had thought to bring me the pineapple and was willing to embrace me was all the proof I required.

I was gutted by a series of complex emotions. I felt like a child, and Sekai reminded me of my mother, who would console me whenever I cried. When was the last time I had cried before today? I couldn't remember, even though the grandmothers had shared so many stories about the therapeutic power of tears. In this moment, with Sekai, I could sense that everything that was present — my anger, my sadness, my hope, my need for consolation — was obvious to Sekai, without me having to utter a word about it. Like any mother, she felt it.

I don't know how long we stood together like that, but eventually, we sat back down. Both of us looked out the same window that Erica had always gazed through as she beheld the guava tree, filled with a chorus of noisy finches. Today, it had no fruits, no leaves, no noisy finches; they had abandoned the tree for their seasonal migration.

"It's so quiet when the guavas aren't in season, isn't it?" Sekai whispered to herself.

Too emotional to make sustained eye contact, I just nodded as I looked at the tree and struggled to find my voice.

Perhaps in an attempt to break the awkward silence, Sekai asked, "How is Resistance?"

"He is doing well," I replied. I was reminded of the fact that this question had once been Erica's unfailing refrain. "I'm so sorry," I finally said, my eyes filling with tears once more.

And as I imagine my mother would have said to me, and as the grandmothers had been saying virtually since I'd met them, Sekai gently offered, "It's OK, my child. It's OK to cry."

The tables had turned. I openly wept, but some part of me still felt embarrassed, as if I were being unprofessional by giving Sekai a window into my own grief. She could sense it. To fill the silence, she said, "I never really asked you about the land of pineapples. I just knew from Nurse Takashinga that you fell in love with pineapples. Do you have stories about your travels in the land of pineapples?"

"It's called Benin." I sniffed.

"Well, that one is from Honde Valley," she said pointing at the pineapple on the desk. "Why don't you tell me a little bit about Benin?" She smiled encouragingly, as if she knew that I needed a distraction from my raw sorrow.

"Ouidah — that was the name of the place."

"So you just went there for the pineapples?" she remarked mischievously.

I had never shared details about my Ouidah experience (not many people had asked about it, either), but there was something about Sekai's piercing yet gentle eyes, paired with my current frail state and desire to jettison the present moment altogether, that allowed my words to flow.

"Sometimes you go to a place, and you experience so much when you leave that place, you have a million questions about yourself, your life. You question things that you once took for granted," I began. I was surprised by the words that were coming out of my mouth, but as soon as I said them, I knew they were true.

"Long ago, people spoke like that about Wenera," Sekai said. "You weren't born yet, so you will not know what Wenera was — it was a journey to a land of gold, a different culture, different singing, and a different language. It brought about much wealth and often much suffering, too."

Actually, I did know about Wenera. It was a term for the gold mines in South Africa; people in the southern part of Africa, such as Zimbabwe, Mozambique, Botswana, and Malawi, would take a train to Wenera. If they came back, they would do so with a substantial amount of money and flashy clothes. The transition from having no money to making a small fortune in Wenera often resulted in the breakup of marriages and families. Many men who left their home countries remained in Wenera for years; sometimes, they married new women and had entirely new families.

"I guess Ouidah was my Wenera, then, but I didn't really suffer when I was there. I just came back with a lot of new insights," I said. "Apart from the pineapples, I experienced voodoo, which challenged some of my views about culture and mental health."

Sekai cocked her head to one side. "What is voodoo?"

I considered the question; I didn't really know if I had a sufficient answer. "It's a religion…maybe a culture? It's a way of life that has defined West Africa and other faraway places associated with the slave trade. I don't know much about it, but the little I picked up has enabled me to appreciate non-Christian culture and religion a lot more," I said. It was absolutely true, since I'd been raised in a staunchly Christian household, by a mother who would never have allowed me to approach voodoo with a ten-foot pole!

"So when you say you experienced voodoo, was this like going to a traditional healer here in Zimbabwe?" Sekai wondered.

I wanted to explain what I understood about voodoo now, but it was challenging. Yes, the healing component was very important, but especially after my work with the grandmothers, I recognized there was something else about the religion that had struck me as unique. When I was in Ouidah, everyone seemed to share a powerful feeling of connection. I couldn't sense any loneliness whatsoever. Everyone was friendly to everyone else, and I could tell from the easy way in which people interacted that there were ineffable threads holding the fabric of their society together.

"No, I think voodoo is more than that," I said. "Voodoo is the oldest religion that was embraced by Africans. It was here before the Christians came. And women play a powerful role in voodoo because the divine creator is a woman."

"Ah!" she exclaimed. "They worship a Mwari [god] who is female?"

"Yes, and that god is called Mawu."

She smiled impishly. "I like that — a female god! OK, so tell me more."

As I told Sekai the story, I found myself traveling back in time to an experience that, unbeknownst to me, would coalesce with the work I was doing with the fourteen grandmothers and forever transform my understanding of the power that is inherent in community-oriented approaches to healing.

During the time I was still seeing Erica as a patient, as I mentioned in chapter 1, I was invited to attend a World Health Organization meeting on mental health legislation and human rights in Ouidah. The arrivals lounge at Cotonou Cadjehoun Airport was hot and humid. An elegantly dressed middle-aged man in a yellow necktie seemed unperturbed by the heat as he stood calmly reading his book amid the frenzy of arriving passengers scrambling for landing cards.

An air of authority hung over the man in the yellow necktie as he kept a distance from the chaos, his eyes fixed on the pages of his book: *Ma vie* (*My Life*), by Bill Clinton. Soon his status was confirmed by three uniformed men, and he was whisked away to a door labeled VIP.

As I walked out into the late-afternoon heat of Cotonou, a swarm of taxi drivers approached me, jostling for my attention. "Taxi, taxi, mon ami, taxi? Où vas-tu?"

"Non, merci," I replied, putting my best French-speaking foot forward as I scanned the horizon for my cue — a large blue sign with the acronyms OMS/WHO, held by an elderly bearded man I'd been told would be waiting for me.

As I walked toward the man with the sign, I glimpsed the man in the yellow necktie under a shaded terrace, gesticulating passionately and talking into a microphone held by a journalist. A small crowd listened intently while reporters frantically clicked their cameras.

He must be someone important, I thought.

"Dixon?" the man holding the OMS placard inquired.

"Yes," I replied with relief.

"Je m'appelle Azagba," he said, placing his hand on his chest before putting my hand luggage in the back seat of the OMS minibus.

The van's air conditioner offered a welcome relief from the humidity. "Welcome to Cotonou," Azagba began as he drove. "First time…aah, here?" he asked, struggling with his English.

"Oui, c'est ma première fois," I responded, meeting him halfway with my rudimentary French. "Azagba, who is that man with the yellow tie, là-bas?" I pointed in the general direction of the man, who was still speaking in front of several microphones.

"Stupid people — very not good." Azagba's baritone response held a note of irritation. "Politics of Benin — c'est très mal." I decided not to ask any more questions. I had been well informed during the WHO pretravel brief to avoid getting involved in local politics.

However, for Azagba, this was an opportunity to vent his fury at Mr. Yellow Necktie and his type. He launched into a French-English monologue of how a beautiful country was being ruined by the greedy elites. "The French government is part of this problem through their firm control and manipulation of the West African franc!"

After enduring a good hour of Azagba's political discourse on Benin, not to mention his dislike of drivers from Cotonou, we finally arrived at my destination: Ouidah.

The WHO compound in Ouidah was enclosed by an imposingly high perimeter wall. At the entrance, a young man in a security uniform handed Azagba a clipboard with a form to sign and reminded him in the local language, Fulani, that I was not to leave the compound without informing security — WHO protocol to protect the well-being of their visitors. I was put off by the walls that separated the inside from the outside and kept out the villagers. I felt that perhaps I was being insulated from the culture of voodoo that permeated the streets of Ouidah. It seemed contrary to the aims of an organization like the WHO, since public health required understanding of local culture.

While waiting for my room to be set up, I was invited to sit in the canteen and was offered slices of pineapple by the manager, a tall, upright man with scarification on his cheeks — most likely from a coming-of-age ritual, which was common in Benin.

Sitting under a rickety overhead fan for maximum breeze, I took my first mouthful. There's something about a novel taste when it first explodes in your mouth that provides you with an unforgettable experience that can be summoned to mind years later. It's not that I had never tasted pineapples before, but there was something distinctly divine and succulent about this pineapple I was eating.

The canteen manager was looking at me intently and grinning. "Vous êtes de quel pays?"

"Zimbabwe."

He smiled. "Zee best pineapple in Ouidah!"

I nodded approvingly as I continued to savor the peppery-sweet taste and thought to myself, *I could eat this every day!*

"Antiga blaaa," the canteen manager suddenly blurted out, grinning from ear to ear.

"Sorry, my French not good," I mumbled. I must have sounded like I was intoxicated, pineapple juice dribbling from the corner of my mouth.

"Anti-ga blaa-ck," he repeated slowly.

"Antigua black?"

"Oui. Zee best pineapples, most delicious!" He flicked his long fingers in the air. "They come from Antigua, but Ouidah pineapples same as zee Antigua pineapples. Très bon!"

I couldn't agree more as I accepted a second and third helping.

But when you eat something new for the first time, it's easy to overdo it. Later that evening, in my room, I learned that too much pineapple causes diarrhea.

I was still on the toilet seat after taking my second dose of loperamide when the first drumbeat tore through the night sky. The seemingly random sound caught me off guard, but it was nevertheless a welcome distraction from the sound of my bowels.

I wondered if I would be spending the whole night on the toilet. Gentle male voices mumbled in Fulani outside the walls of the compound. Suddenly, a single thunderous beat made up of dozens of djembe drums resounded through the darkness.

It was not a restful night, but fortunately, the loperamide worked.

The next day, after I was introduced to other delegates from several countries, I took the opportunity to talk to Azagba and ask him about the all-night drum orchestra that had kept me awake.

"Vaudou, mon ami, c'est le vaudou ici à Ouidah," he said with a mischievous smile.

I picked up the French word for *voodoo* but nothing beyond that. Fortunately, my Ghanaian colleague, who had a better grasp of French, came to the rescue while holding a plate of sliced pineapple. Watching him attack his fourth helping, I thought to myself, *It's just a matter of time!*

I also thought about what Azagba had said. I knew next to nothing about voodoo. Growing up in the harsh environment of an urban township, my mother would instruct my siblings and me to stay away from things we didn't know. But my paternal grandmother, the one whom we'd visit in the khips, would encourage us to explore the world. She insisted, "Little knowledge is poison." During the 1930s she was one of the few educated Black women in Rhodesia, able to read and write. She was also fiercely independent and strong-willed — she'd left her first husband to marry my grandfather, a move considered heretical by both the colonial governors and her native Karanga clan.

What little I did know of voodoo was probably poisoned by stereotypes and misunderstandings. Despite its African roots, my perception of the religion was abstract and probably unduly Hollywood influenced, less connected to the rhythmic drums I'd heard the night before and more to White colonialist ideas about the "savage" or "evil" aspects of African culture. My mother, sadly, would probably have agreed. "The devil is manipulative and enticing," she might have said.

"You don't do pineapples?" my Ghanaian colleague quipped, interrupting my thoughts.

"I overdid it last night. I got sick after feasting on pineapples," I explained, slightly embarrassed.

"You got sick from pineapple?" He laughed. "You don't have pineapples in Zimbabwe?"

I shrugged as we walked into the auditorium, semi-wondering how I might be able to have my fill of pineapple again without crossing over into sickness.

In the workshop, we focused on the human rights of people with mental disorders in Africa. At lunch five of us sat around a well-polished wooden table discussing WHO's ten basic principles of mental healthcare law. A spirited colleague from Malawi argued that these principles ignored the need for adequate financial and human resources to implement them.

While we ate, I casually inquired about voodoo. Each person had a different opinion. One was quick to dismiss the superstitious nature of voodoo. "These people believe in voodoo dolls," he said with disdain, "like they can control you remotely using a doll." He laughed and waved a hand, dismissing the mere thought. Another colleague was cautious and advised me to talk to the locals if I wanted to know more.

We changed the subject back to our original talking points. As we exchanged our thoughts about mentally ill people, who were routinely tied to trees and kept in captivity in the most inhumane ways, my thoughts kept flitting back to the drums. I wondered if Azagba might be the right person to give me the details I wanted — about both pineapples and voodoo.

The early evenings in Ouidah brought the refreshing, salty smell of the Atlantic Ocean into the compound, along with the sound of the rising tides. The mosquitoes were out with a vengeance and made it impossible to venture outdoors without multiple applications of mosquito repellent. I was glad to be sitting in the canteen after a long first day, listening to the canteen manager talk to local delegates in Fulani. I joined two locals, who were sipping cold local coconut water from Coke Is Great drinking glasses, and asked them if there were any sightseeing or fun activities they recommended in Ouidah for a first-timer like myself.

The younger of the two people was eager to share his knowledge. "You can go out on a tour with local guides, or you can walk out on your own, but you have to be careful not to get lost or be taken advantage of by the locals," he advised.

The older man, who had a little white beard, intervened. "You'll have no problem — it's actually quite safe."

"What about the voodoo?" I asked, trying to sound nonchalant. "What's it all about?"

"Voodoo is the way of life here. There's a big annual meeting currently running, so you will hear drums most evenings," the older man explained.

"Can I go see the drumming?"

"Yes, but it's best to go with local people," he said.

"No, you don't need local people," the young one piped up before giving in to the older man's insistence on an escort. "Oui, oui, c'est vrai."

By the third day of my trip, I was excited that I was able to eat pineapples again! I'd also managed to get a good idea of what was happening outside the walls of the WHO compound. From my chat with Azagba and a handful of others, I had put together a rough mental sketch of the city. I had also managed to collect some information about a few important matters. Namely, I discovered that in 1996, voodoo was declared a national religion in Benin by President Nicéphore Soglo.

According to Azagba, when President Mathieu Kérékou took office in 1996, during his swearing-in ceremony, he forgot to reference the voodoo spirits, and there was such an outcry that he was forced to return and take the oath once more.

Despite the fact that voodoo had been around for a very long time, I found few positive references about it; mostly, I encountered screeds that decried it as a religion centered on "black magic." Was it truly so evil? The rhythmic djembe drums that tore through the night sky had been celebratory and sounded anything but evil.

Azagba connected me to a young mechanic named Mamoudou, who was willing to be my guide for a modest fee of ten dollars. Mamoudou had a good grasp of English, which he'd acquired during his training as a mechanic in Nigeria. Over a local dish of *fufu* and fish *yassa*, Mamoudou began the journey of enlightening me: "The highest power in voodoo is a woman, an elder woman — usually a mother who is gentle, loving, and forgiving. She is also considered as the god who is above all other gods, and even if there is no temple or worshipping shrine made in her name, the people pray to her, especially in times of distress. You know, Haiti became the first free Black republic because of voodoo. The slaves revolted, and what unified them was the spirit of voodoo."

I listened intently, unable to tell how much of what I heard was indeed fact.

Mamoudou told me that syncretism, the amalgamation of different religious and cultural practices, arose on the continent "because people like you and me, Black people, were not allowed by colonizers to worship their own gods"; rather, they were forced into worshipping the Christian god. But, like many oppressed people, they found a way around this injunction by using Christianity and the church as an entry point into their own spiritual traditions.

There was something else he said that caught my attention: "The seeds of Black revolt against slavery were planted by voodoo, whether in Haiti, in South America, or even in the southern parts of the USA. It was voodoo, and that is why it's deliberately portrayed as an evil, primitive lifestyle — but the thing to remember is that the core root of voodoo is freedom." I couldn't help but make an indirect association with Resistance. Perhaps his eccentric name had a deeper meaning and purpose.

"Voodoo philosophy is very closely linked to nature," Mamoudou emphasized. According to him, it was not possible to kill voodoo or to outlaw it altogether because it was in all of us, and it had been for a long time. He spent a considerable amount of time talking about the slave revolt that ultimately freed the island of Haiti, making it the first truly Black republic in the world.

"You ever heard of the Underground Railroad in the US?" he asked.

It sounded familiar, but I didn't know much about it.

"Strong voodoo influence and rituals that guided the slaves to the free world!" affirmed Mamoudou, nodding his head. He also informed me that Benin had existed as the kingdom of Dahomey well before the Europeans came to Africa — and, furthermore, that women had been part of the military, since Dahomey was an egalitarian society in many respects.

"An all-female military regiment was the characteristic feature of the army of Dahomey," he said with a smile. "But these people say we ill treat our women. Voodoo has always respected the African woman — that is why, my brother, it is feared by the Western world. Voodoo is too strong!"

I appreciated that Mamoudou had a deep grasp of his culture...or was he just a good tour guide? I didn't know how I felt about what he was saying, but I politely listened, eager to learn more. A story is only as good as its storyteller, and Mamoudou was a great storyteller who never failed to transport me to different worlds and vantage points, many of which would stay with me during the daytime WHO convenings.

After several days of experiencing life outside the walls of the WHO compound, it became apparent to me that there was a disconnect between what locals believed and what we were discussing in our workshop about human rights. The stated ideals around human rights, as lofty and noble as they sounded, were completely disengaged from the rich cultural heritage of the place where we were located. It felt like such a missed opportunity. The culture and history of Ouidah were oozing out of every structure beyond our walls.

One evening, Mamoudou took me to his house for a meal. He introduced me to his wife and two children, then we ate a local fish dish with cassava. After the meal, he told me, "I've secured a slot for us to attend the priestess's healing ceremony." We headed down a dusty path to meet a voodoo priestess at a local village shrine. I'd been curious about traditional ceremonies ever since Mamoudou had regaled me with stories about this esteemed and ancient religion. Our walk brought back memories of my own childhood, back when shoes were a luxury. It seemed so normal to walk around barefoot then... how the world had changed! I reminisced about the simple pleasures of that time as I walked alongside Mamoudou between mango and banana trees.

The temple was a rondavel, a traditional African circular building with a thatched roof. Numerous pieces of paraphernalia hung from the roof, and chicken feathers of different sizes were tied to a wooden, phallus-like object hanging from the central beam. On the floor lay several containers with lids on them. One of them was embellished with what appeared to be a crocodile skull; on another was a human skull. I couldn't take my eyes off the human skull.

Mamoudou noticed my fixation and said, "The skull belongs to an ancestor of the priestess."

I raised a skeptical eyebrow. "Mamoudou, you are full of shit, my brother!"

"No, seriously," he whispered. "Voodoo is passed on from family to family. In voodoo, we worship our ancestors, and we believe that the spirits of the dead live side by side with the living."

According to Mamoudou, every family has its own female priesthood, which is sometimes hereditary if the lineage moves from mother to daughter.

The voodoo priestess, an elderly woman who appeared to be in her seventies, kept a calm demeanor as she attended to the many people who came to see her. I was specifically interested in watching her conduct healings linked to suspected mental illness, or what the locals referred to as spiritually related illness. A number of people came on that particular day. I witnessed the healing of what may have been epilepsy in an adolescent. I was told the young man had been brought in because he had experienced what was described as a seizure the previous day, and he was now showing signs of confusion. Of course, there was no way of verifying any of this. The priestess seemed to hypnotize the young boy through her soft incantations until he fell into a deep sleep.

I was also struck by her interaction with a young woman who had what seemed to be postpartum depression; she didn't say any of this, but I assumed it on the basis of what she shared with the priestess. The priestess started by asking the young mother to talk about her life. The woman described how she had struggled with sleep, fatigue, and feeling detached from her newborn baby. At some point, the priestess took the baby, who was crying out in irritation, in her arms and rocked the little one. As she spoke gentle words to the mother, she gazed at the baby in the most loving and empathetic way until he quieted down, giving only the occasional contented murmur.

I noticed that the priestess seemed to have a similar magic touch with others, as well as the capacity to respond masterfully to whatever was happening in the room with a mere change in the tone of her voice or a shift in her body language. More than any of my other experiences in Ouidah, my time with the voodoo priestess was the most profound.

It seemed from my brief encounter with her that what one did for a living was altogether irrelevant. The reason people had gone to her to be healed was perhaps less about the magical properties of voodoo and more about the space she'd created for people to tell their stories. Obviously, the woman was not a Western-trained therapist or psychiatrist, but she had the uncanny ability to respond to each person with the quality of unadulterated attention and care.

I didn't know if I was walking away from my encounters in Ouidah with a comprehensive picture of voodoo — in both its historical and its social implications for African people — but

I did know that my eyes were opened to something very valuable. Voodoo was about relationships, about reaching out to each other and touching the humanness that is in each one of us. As Mamoudou had already affirmed, voodoo was about connection with self, other, and spirit.

"Might this not be what each one of us is striving for in our own unique ways as we look for purpose in our lives and communities?" I mused aloud later when I shared my story with Sekai. "I come from a Christian background, but being immersed in voodoo didn't feel frightening or threatening. It was humbling. I started to ask myself why voodoo is considered evil when it has this much love coursing through it."

Sitting there with Sekai, I remembered talking to the grandmothers about my experience in Ouidah. I had told them that I believed what I'd encountered was a higher level of consciousness — and that what had struck me the most was the singing, the dancing, and the rhythmic drumming, which would rise and fall and rise again into a crescendo. There was nothing about the experience that felt chaotic or turbulent. All of it was perfectly choreographed, a way of sending people into a deep trance state that would calm their nerves and help them to heal from whatever was holding them back.

Once, I had described this encounter to Grandmother Jack. She simply nodded and affirmed, "There is no culture that is superior to another culture." I knew that she was right. Voodoo had been assailed by unwarranted contempt and superstition, not to mention attitudes of blatant racism and false ideas of cultural supremacy, but it had great wisdom to share with all of us.

In the midst of my conversation with Sekai, we were interrupted by the clinic nurse, who reminded me that it was time to go. As we stood up to leave, Sekai said, "It seems like you got something very valuable in Ouidah — more than just your love of pineapples!"

I laughed, feeling a new sense of ease with her after crying my heart out and sharing a story I'd told only a few others. "There is so much about voodoo I still don't understand. I have tried to read about it, and there are often conflicting narratives. But I think the idea of the goddess being an elderly woman, usually a mother who is gentle and forgiving, is quite nurturing and helpful. And it feels true to me."

Sekai sighed. "Do you think things would have been different if we'd taken Erica to a traditional healer in our village when we couldn't find money to come here?"

"I don't know," I responded. "I think there's room for communities to play a more active role. I'm currently working with fourteen grandmothers in Mbare to try and help those in need of emotional support to have a first port of call in their community. I've learned a lot from them. I think if Erica and other people in distress had more people like the grandmothers in their communities — people to go to immediately in times of need — it would be better for everyone."

"Maybe," Sekai said. "Maybe someday you could consider me as one of your grandmothers on your project and I could help my community in Mutare."

"What a great idea! I would love that," I replied.

"Maybe if I had been trained, I would have seen it coming with Erica and I would have acted before she did it." She paused to reflect. "I'm telling you, Doctor, I really thought she was not doing too badly — that we could wait until we had enough money to come and see you. She seemed very active the few days before she took her own life. She went up the mango tree every day to read her book." She stopped suddenly as tears began to flow down her face. "I came to the garden to call her to come inside to have her lunch, and I saw her hanging from the tree."

That recollection was enough for Sekai to erupt into sobs. Nurse Takashinga heard the sobbing and came in. Neither of us said anything. Nurse Takashinga simply put her arm around Sekai's shoulder. We all stood there with her as she wept. Sadness welled inside me, too, but this time, I managed not to cry.

After she calmed down, Sekai turned to me and asked, "Can I visit you again?"

"I would love that." We needed each other, at least for now.

For the next three years, Sekai would periodically show up during my Thursday clinic day, always with a pineapple or two. In exchange, I would share more about Ouidah and my excitement about the Friendship Bench as it gained traction. The growing friendship was one I welcomed. Sekai's capacity for listening, her gentle wisdom and humor, belied the fact that she had undergone a tremendous loss — perhaps the greatest loss a person can imagine. But similarly to the grandmothers, and perhaps to the voodoo priestess I'd encountered in Benin, it had equipped her with a specific resilience and compassion that marks all those who've lived through tremendous suffering but who've managed to keep their hearts open.

I recognized that we were engaged in the kind of mutual healing that the Friendship Bench, with its focus on the power of community, was proving to be a necessary part of a life well lived. What was more, I had the sense that the key to healing lay in all the hidden treasures within African cultures — which I'd witnessed firsthand on that trip to Benin, where I'd fallen under the spell of pineapples and voodoo — and that these treasures might help us transmute the suffering that seemed to infuse our individual and collective story.

For this, I was beyond grateful.

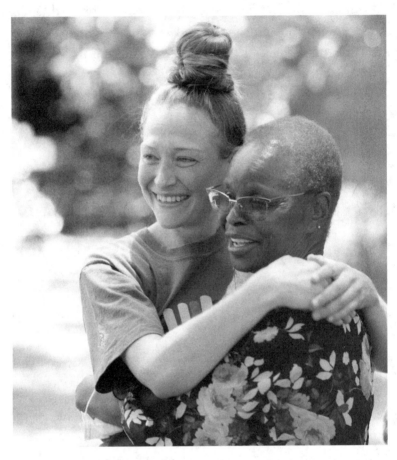

Grandmother Kusi with Friendship Bench program designer Jean Turner, one of the humblest people I have had the opportunity to work with. Over the ten years I've worked with her, her dedication and commitment to the values of Friendship Bench have always been unwavering.

Chapter Five

Resistance

M y conversation with Sekai and my reminiscences about the encounter with the voodoo priestess in Benin reminded me of the almost prophetic words of my tour guide, Mamoudou: "The highest power in voodoo is a woman, an elder woman — usually a mother who is gentle, loving, and forgiving. She is also considered as the god who is above all other gods, and even if there is no temple or worshipping shrine made in her name, the people pray to her, especially in times of distress."

Indeed, maternal comfort had been a healing balm — not just for me since that cathartic meeting with Sekai that led to our sustained friendship, but also for the many people in my city who were reeling from the aftermath of civil unrest. It seemed that the gifts of our grandmothers, which had been extolled across the continent for eons, were not just ancestral relics, but medicine that was desperately needed in the times in which we found ourselves.

By 2007, nearly two years after Erica's death, the Friendship Bench initiative, helmed by fourteen wise and opinionated grandmothers, had gained enormous popularity in the community of Mbare. The first conspicuous sign of this was that people outside of Mbare, from other areas of the city of Harare, had begun to come to the bench to receive wise counsel from the grandmothers. Often, these people would go back to their communities and discuss the need for a Friendship Bench in their own vicinity.

Word spread like wildfire about the service that the grandmothers were providing, and the wheels of inspiration began to turn. Just as Sekai had suggested to me during our first meeting after Erica's death, there were many who wondered if grandmothers in their own communities could provide the same service. City authorities got wind of this, and the idea of introducing the Friendship Bench to all the communities of Harare circulated in no time.

Of course, it would take a few more years before the Friendship Bench received the kind of generous funding that would truly support a citywide initiative to train grandmothers in even more neighborhoods, as Harare was still financially strapped, but the political will behind our work gave us the impetus to continue and to see where it would all eventually go.

Our initial measurements of who had been served by the fourteen grandmothers were not exactly accurate, since, at this stage, we were much more concerned with the caliber of support we were providing than with the more clinical metrics, such as the DSM and ICD-10, that the grandmothers had derided from the outset. We ended up surmising that around thirty thousand people had been served by the Friendship Bench within the first few years — a tenfold increase from the grandmothers' work in our first few months!

We continued to consider more ways we could leverage everything we'd already done so that we could help the greatest number of people possible. One day about two years into the start of the Friendship Bench, Grandmother Jack adjusted her red beret against the morning sun and gave me an earnest look. "Now listen, Doctor — as you know, the first thing we do when a client sits on the bench is kuvhura pfungwa," opening the mind.

An enthusiastic chorus of "Hongu" followed from the other grandmothers.

"That training in problem-solving therapy that we had when we first started is a good foundation," Grandmother Jack continued. "And also the ongoing refresher training and supervision from Nurse Shelly."

Nurse Shelly had been a godsend to our intrepid group of elders. Although the nurses at the clinic in Mbare had been much too busy to provide the grandmothers with supervision, as I'd initially hoped they would, I'd managed to get a modest grant to bring Nurse Shelly on board on a part-time basis to train the grandmothers, as my responsibilities at the hospital meant I could not be a constant presence.

Grandmother Jack sat back in her chair, her arms crossed against her chest as she gazed thoughtfully into space. "But the truth is, there are more essential concerns at play here." She looked for reinforcement from the others, who nodded in agreement. I could tell they'd all discussed this prior to our meeting.

"The way the community actually views mental health

or mental illness should be what drives the Friendship Bench — not the so-called books." She pointed out that we needed a holistic approach that brought into consideration the socioeconomic challenges people were facing. "And we need to involve the community in a much bigger way." She readjusted her red beret, as if for dramatic effect. "This is why I think we should work with Resistance more intentionally."

When Resistance was readmitted to my hospital, sometime after Erica's death and the formation of the Friendship Bench initiative, I had decided to introduce him to the grandmothers, who I felt could provide additional support and would be there for Resistance whenever he needed to talk. While he certainly seemed to feel at home in the hospital, he lacked anything that felt like sustainable support — and though the people who worked at the hospital were kind enough to him, I was beginning to realize that kindness wasn't enough. The grandmothers had opened my eyes (as well as my mind and heart) to the importance of community, to the human need for a deeper connection with people who have the capacity to hold space for suffering while reminding us of the fact that we are much more than our suffering — and that poverty is a state of mind that, with the help of necessary perspective and reflection and despite historical injustices and constrained resources, we can actually transcend.

After a brainstorming session about Resistance's needs, I had selected Grandmother Jack to be his one-on-one point person. Their relationship inevitably led to a drop in Resistance's readmission rate. Beyond this, we gained valuable insider information about the specifics of Resistance's living conditions; while the hospital was aware of what he'd had to endure, Grandmother Jack had garnered even more details about the level of abuse Resistance was subjected to on a daily basis from neighbors who'd labeled him a madman.

Before meeting with me, the grandmothers had unanimously determined that Resistance needed more than just counseling or medication; he needed psychosocial support, which would come from meaningful social interaction and a sense of acceptance from not just the grandmothers but his own community. Conveniently, Resistance lived in Mbare, where the Friendship Bench was located.

"Resistance is a troubled soul." Grandmother Jack sighed. "But things might change for the better moving forward."

As was her way, Grandmother Jack had asked Resistance to offer his take on what was happening and what might help improve his social interactions. He had suggested, "What about groups meeting regularly to talk about the community and how they can help each other?" I was impressed by the suggestion, as well as by Grandma Jack's shrewdness in empowering Resistance to offer his own solutions to the problem at hand.

"We could encourage people at the bench to join community support groups," Grandmother Jack enthusiastically told us. "These same people could then invite others in their community, and they could collectively problem solve around common issues. It would be a collective opening of the mind!"

"It's a good example of not just focusing on a single approach," agreed Grandmother Hwiza. "Because we're not convinced that Resistance actually needs medication!"

I was intrigued by some of the grandmothers' suggestions on how to help Resistance. When I'd first met him, he was already part of the psychiatric unit, as his diagnosis had been made four years before I joined the hospital staff. Because he'd been on medication for a while, it was hard for me to establish what his state had been prior to this.

At the same time, I wasn't convinced that the medication was making much of a difference in terms of his quality of life. After all, whenever he came to the hospital with a relapse, he didn't really display the common symptoms of schizophrenia. In fact, Resistance's first admission to the hospital was due to a substance-induced psychosis. When this occurs, a patient doesn't need to be put on medication for the rest of their life; in fact, medication should be used only to contain the psychosis. After this, if they refrain from substances altogether, they should be fine. However, this had not been the case with Resistance. He'd been placed on continuous medication with only a few "drug holidays," during which he seemed to do quite well. The grandmothers had intuitively picked up on the possibility that we could take Resistance off medication altogether.

Grandmother Chizhande said, "He probably doesn't even have schizophrenia. We know that when young men smoke *mbanje* [cannabis], they can go mad. Resistance told us that he was admitted to the psychiatric unit after a period of serious cannabis smoking, and then they gave him a monthly injection. And then, on top of that, he was given haloperidol [an antipsychotic], and when he started shaking from the side effects, the entire community was convinced he was mad!"

"And with a name like Resistance, all he had to do was play the part," quipped Grandmother Jack.

Grandmother Kusi offered, "Resistance's story is of a man who has struggled to find a partner, friends, and a sense of community because of the stigma he has had to live with." The others nodded compassionately.

According to the grandmothers, Resistance had found solace in the psychiatric hospital, but he didn't really belong in a "madhouse," as Grandmother Jack put it. He needed community acceptance, above all.

Thus, the Friendship Bench expanded; it was no longer just a one-on-one service offered on a park bench. Now the grandmothers were determined to provide more in-depth community support.

Knowledge is power — and it also ensures a more connected and responsive community. Two weeks after our debriefing session, Grandmother Jack, Grandmother Hwiza, Grandmother Kusi, and Grandmother Chizhande went to the area where Resistance lived and knocked on doors. Their goal was to sensitize the neighborhood about mental illness and why some people may show madness (psychosis) after taking cannabis; they emphasized that these people, including Resistance, could be helped. They brought a much-needed message of tough love and community cohesion, to which people attentively listened. The grandmothers were particularly clever when it came to connecting the dots between good mental health and the capacity to address the numerous problems the residents faced: clean drinking water and access to healthcare, to name a couple. Perhaps more expertly than any public health official, the grandmothers were able to drive home the point that caring for our mental health is what enables us to pool our minds and resources together and come up with solutions for seemingly insurmountable challenges. It helped that they weren't strangers, but highly respected community members who acted as harbingers of hope for everyone they encountered.

The community visits had emerged from the wisdom of Grandmother Chizhande, who seemed to be especially focused on raising mental health awareness in pragmatic ways. "We need to go to these houses and let people know there is nothing unusual about Resistance," she said. "He's not possessed by evil spirits, and he's not a madman — he's just struggling with the issues a lot of people struggle with. If we let people know that he simply needs to connect with others and he isn't going to hurt anyone, change is possible."

I'd come to the same realization during my first several interactions with Resistance. He had no interest in hurting anyone; he was simply starved for connection and understanding. However, while my observation was shared among the hospital staff, Grandmother Chizhande was onto something important: Resistance's situation could change for the better only if the people in his community recognized his deeper need for connection. Although the grandmothers' idea to visit his community was not some kind of sophisticated intervention, this impetus to touch base with so many people seemed remarkable to me. It could be a way to get to one of the root causes of Resistance's malaise: being subject to loneliness and misunderstanding.

Aside from the community visits, the peer support groups Resistance had suggested — which we eventually called Circle Kubatana Tose (meaning "holding hands together" in Shona, as I mentioned in the preface) — began in earnest shortly after my debriefing conversation with the grandmothers. The first group had ten members, including Resistance. Unsurprisingly, with the combination of community education being provided by both the grandmothers and the first peer group, which was facilitated primarily by Grandmother Jack, Resistance's readmission rate fell even further.

I realized that just as Resistance had found a sense of purpose at the hospital through his "helper" duties, the peer group served a similar function. It made him feel that he truly belonged. The group had a circle format (which my own wise maternal grandmother had suggested during one of our conversations about the Friendship Bench); the members sat in a circle and passed a talking stick around. Whoever held the talking stick had the opportunity to speak uninterrupted, with the attention of the group entirely on them. Resistance had never been given the opportunity to talk in such an open way and, moreover, to feel that others were really listening.

Aside from the efficacy of the talking stick — some form of which is well-known in most traditional and Indigenous communities around the world, and which has been adopted by Westerners in everything from restorative justice circles to organizational retreats — the peer group also took turns brainstorming ways to address individuals' specific problems. It was a level of support that boosted Resistance's morale and made him feel that he was valued.

Later on, Grandmother Jack shared, "When he joined that group, he began to thrive. And it's not because of the medication — it's the companionship and acceptance he's getting from a community of people who care about him."

I was overjoyed to see that the grandmothers' suggestions were bearing fruit in the community. In general, they were the ones who ultimately determined whether someone needed more in-depth support (in the form of community visits or peer group participation) based on the severity of the challenge they were facing. For example, if a woman was a victim of intimate partner violence, she would be assigned to a grandmother who would then provide her with more one-on-one support. This could include moving the woman to a shelter or being available on call in case of a crisis. Often, the grandmothers determined whether someone was at risk if they scored high on the SSQ screening tool and it was clear that they required greater attention and focus.

The point of their work, ultimately, was to ensure that no one who came to the Friendship Bench ever felt that they had to walk through their troubles alone. Empowering patients was paramount in this work, but as the grandmothers understood, empowerment was part and parcel of being among people who believed in you and who would be with you every step of the way.

I was fascinated to see how the grandmothers processed the different steps of the therapy that they provided, which went beyond the training they had received and encompassed their combined thousand years of wisdom and life experience. Over time, I began to identify a specific pattern at work. First, the grandmothers focused on a challenge that the client was undergoing during their initial session. Once a person's mind was open, "it's like you now have space to unpack that problem without the clutter of all the other problems," explained Grandmother Chinhoyi.

After kuvhura pfungwa, the next step was kusimudzira

(uplifting the client), which entailed hand-holding and giving someone the motivation and tools that were necessary to tackle what they were going through headfirst.

"Sometimes you have this problem," explained Grandmother Mako. "For example, I talked with a mother who has no money for her daughter's school fees, and she is totally beside herself seeing her nine-year-old crying each morning because she can't go to school with the other kids. Then, the mother begins to worry about the daughter and everything else that is already going wrong: a husband who is a waste of time, a four-year-old son who is showing signs of malnutrition, the eviction letter that has been sitting on the kitchen table for three weeks, the last time they had a proper meal. Doctor, it can be endless, the list of things going wrong for people here." She paused. "When I listened to her story and summarized the things she was struggling with, she looked at me and burst into tears once more —"

Grandmother Jack interrupted, looking pointedly at me. "By the way, we really need to have tissues on hand, because people cry a lot on the bench!"

Grandmother Mako nodded. "Yes, that's true! Anyway, she cried, and she couldn't decide which problem to address first. After we prayed together, she settled down and said, 'I want my child at school because when she is at school, I can deal with the other problems.'"

"What did she mean?" I inquired.

"Well, she said something that shocked me: 'If my child is at home on her own, I can't go out looking for income, because if I leave her alone, I worry her stepfather will sexually abuse her.' At that, she broke down and cried some more."

"Men can be dogs," muttered Grandmother Chinhoyi.

The grandmothers nodded, as if they'd momentarily forgotten that a man was in their midst.

Grandmother Mako continued, "So that's one example of a situation that someone might bring to the bench. The uplifting process happens when we can reassure a client and help them come up with a plan." As Grandmother Mako shared with us, she and the woman figured out how to raise money for her daughter's school fees: the woman would go to the local lake to buy fish, and then she'd resell the fish in her village.

The collective chorus of "Hongu" came once again.

"You know, Doctor," Grandmother Kusi said, "for us, when we talk about uplifting a client, it's not just about helping them identify a problem to work on — it's also about using their language to give them hope."

"Can you give me an example?" I asked.

"Well, let's say you're working with a client who is very religious. I will pray with them using all the pillars of the grandmothers' work, but most of all, I use language that person knows. I had an experience with a young mother who was orphaned at twelve and grew up with no family." The mother was referred to Grandmother Kusi by the clinic nurse because she seemed to be struggling with her emotions. She scored ten on the SSQ and was thinking of harming herself and her two-month-old baby.

"Her main issues were that her baby cried all night and her husband came home drunk every other day," she said. "Of course, she was sad and crying most of the time, and she hated her baby, which made her feel guilty. The Ping-Pong went on for some time. I was surprised that the problem she decided to focus on was her baby's colic. When we started to explore solutions to the colic, she said she was trying to get money to buy gripe water."

Gripe water is a liquid supplement that includes herbs and sodium bicarbonate. Although some mothers will give it to their infants, it's known that giving a baby anything other than breast milk during the first few months of their life can be dangerous and increase the potential for allergies and the introduction of bacteria. The grandmothers chuckled and commented that the poor young mother had been overly indoctrinated into a Western way of thinking by believing that gripe water was good for her baby.

Grandmother Kusi continued, "I had to show her what to do when you have a baby who has colic. This girl had never been taught these things!"

"Young mothers these days now need to be taught how to make their own babies burp," said Grandmother Chinhoyi, laughing. "They don't have that link to the elders who can show them what to do. And if you don't teach these basics, they become suicidal because they can't sleep!"

"This gripe water business is a real problem in the community," Grandmother Jack added. "These people don't realize that it actually has a lot of alcohol — the same as in a bottle of Castle Lager. It's the alcohol that makes the babies sleep! Can you imagine? Giving babies alcohol!"

Grandmother Kusi went on. "So this young mother scored high on the SSQ, but from that one session, after she learned how to make her baby burp, her baby slept peacefully. That meant *she* also slept, so then she could focus on her other issues! So, you see, there is no need to have six sessions with everybody who sits on this bench. Those SSQ scores just mean there's an ongoing challenge, and when you talk to people, you come to understand them on their own terms."

(After that conversation with the grandmothers, I looked for information about the efficacy of single-session therapy. Much to my surprise, I learned it was an entire modality that was thriving in Australia and New Zealand but hadn't quite made it to other parts of the world. The grandmothers had figured out what many Western practitioners hadn't yet realized!)

"When would you say the critical shift occurs once you are interacting with a client?" I asked.

"We see a lot of people who are suicidal here," said Grandmother Nhengo, who was the most educated of the fourteen elders, with three full years of secondary education. "People who respond yes to the SSQ question on suicidal thoughts often have a big shift."

Grandmother Kusi added, "Yes, that's true. And the shift from suicidal thoughts to 'Life is worth it, and I can try again' depends on how well we immerse ourselves in their story. Making people feel respected and understood requires total immersion in their story. That is what we mean when we talk about kuvhura pfungwa. It's a two-way process — and both the client and the grandmother experience this opening of the mind!"

"What is the difference between this opening of the mind and the training you've gone through?" I asked, thinking back to the first order of business when it came to educating the grandmothers on how to provide care to clients who came to the Friendship Bench. From all appearances, it seemed that the grandmothers had mined more gold from their interactions with patients, not to mention from their accumulated years of commonsense wisdom, than from the training they'd received.

True to form, Grandmother Jack boldly replied, "Doctor, you know the PST [problem-solving therapy] approach is mechanical! When someone shows up at the Friendship Bench, you don't just jump into PST. The first thing you say is, 'I'm here for you. Would you like to share your story with me?'" She smiled and added, a bit more gently, "People are not machines. You must remove your medical hat and immerse yourself in the community and their cultural thinking!"

"Sometimes, a client comes here with a score of eleven, and because of protocol, we have to refer them to Nurse Shelly when they have such a high score," said Grandmother Mako. "But we've all learned that even the person with the high score needs to feel like they belong before they're referred to someone else. Because if you panic and immediately refer a person who is suicidal, you could actually make them believe their negative ideas about themselves even more!"

"Again, sharing stories is an important part of this process," affirmed Grandmother Kusi. "Often, when they sense your empathy, they are able to come up with a solution on their own — kind of like Resistance did!"

"Poverty is not always the problem," Grandmother Jack noted. "Often, it is the inability to open our mind that's the problem!"

"We are all poor here in Mbare, but others have double poverty: material and mind poverty," Grandmother Hwiza mused. "They do random things without thinking!"

"Kunge kufungira mumoyo rwendo rwembwa!" Grandmother Jack exclaimed. This is another common Shona idiom that roughly translates as, "The journey of a dog does not require planning." In Harare, you can see many stray dogs wandering around, with no destination in mind. As the saying demonstrates, people can act similarly, engaging in random behavior without thinking through the consequences beforehand.

"People need to think through things, but if everything around you stops you from doing that, then you are climbing a steep hill," added Grandmother Kusi.

Grandmother Mako nodded before moving on to explain the next step in the Friendship Bench process of working with clients. "Finally, there's kusimbisa [strengthening]. This is where we are trying to stop this double poverty mindset." According to the grandmothers, kusimbisa, the third pillar in their process of providing care, offered a way of finding purpose in daily activities, even in the face of seemingly insurmountable obstacles. This was the fuel that gave everyday people the strength to go on — and, even more, to believe they could actually transform their circumstances.

I was impressed that, together, the grandmothers had developed a powerful set of pillars for describing and approaching the therapeutic process. Over time, I felt that I was learning more and more about the efficacy of their approach. Through our conversations, I came to appreciate their sophisticated understanding of what was required for a client to heal and grow beyond their perceived limitations.

Certainly, the grandmothers didn't always agree about everything. In fact, I could remember a number of instances when they vehemently disagreed about certain topics — from whether or not a woman should tell her partner that she was HIV positive to how advisable it was for a client to remain in her home after facing several instances of intimate partner violence. But through these spirited discussions, they always managed to reach a consensus or, at the very least, a respectful compromise. And more often than not, the combination of their voices — from loud and insistent to quiet and steady — created something far greater than the sum of its parts: a philosophy of care that was guided by a deep and powerful desire to do the right thing and to bring every single person they spoke with into the loving fold of a community who saw and appreciated the very best in them.

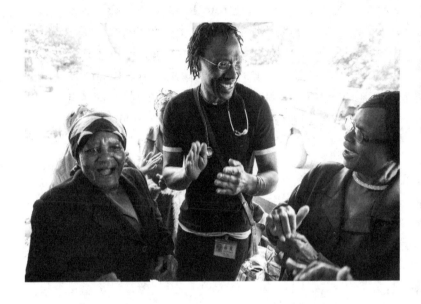

Singing and dancing with the grandmothers during a morning debriefing.

Chapter Six

Songs of Healing, Songs of Grief

More than two very full years had passed since I'd met the wonderfully wise, extremely opinionated, and generously dedicated grandmothers of the Friendship Bench. They had become more than just my friends, colleagues, and mentees — in many ways, they were my true teachers.

My life as a psychiatrist had not allowed me to be so deeply rooted in the larger community of Harare, as I often spent long hours at the hospital attending to patients and the relentless administrative work that is a large part of being one of a small handful of medical professionals in my specific field. But as I spent time with the grandmothers, learning about their lives and going on site visits to the community in Mbare, I was touched by the depth of their care for the people around them, which I was able to see firsthand.

Often, when I was at the clinic in Mbare, I would watch from a distance as the grandmothers offered sessions to community members. Sometimes, with a client's permission, we would also randomly record audio of the sessions on the Friendship Bench, so that we could evaluate programmatic fidelity — meaning we measured the extent to which our intervention was following the model we'd set forth. Such evaluations are always extremely important when it comes to developing an effective model and implementing an evidence-based program, and indeed they would prove to be so in the near future.

I was touched by the willingness of the grandmothers to reveal their own vulnerability. I could see how this melted their clients' reservations, how the clients' tightness and even embarrassment often gave way to laughter, to tears, to the joy of recognizing that they were understood and cared for. The grandmothers had a way of establishing a rapport, a therapeutic alliance, that was like nothing I'd ever seen before — except, perhaps, in the single voodoo ceremony I had been fortunate to witness.

It was not merely their sense of responsibility to their community that propelled their work; for them, it was the only way they'd ever lived and breathed: in connection to everyone around them. This was as true for their pain and sorrow as for their joy and laughter. While I had adopted a more Western way of thinking about people in relation to life — as atomized parts of an always fragmented whole — the grandmothers recognized something that the world at large is now beginning to see and honor: we are all connected, and if we don't realize this soon enough, our persistent sense of isolation might tear us apart.

I began to apply this lesson in my daily psychiatric work and also in my regular interactions with people, trying to be present in the moment. This made me a lot more open to culturally rooted perceptions of well-being and mental health that were an alternative to Western approaches. During my travels, whether I was in Brazil or China or any of the other places where I was increasingly journeying to share the Friendship

Bench model, I observed how people actually interacted with one another in the favelas or the villages and among the Indigenous peoples, who often had their own sophisticated approaches to connection and social cohesion. Although I had favored Western models of care for so long, working with the grandmothers helped me to see where these models were limited — and where my own blind spots were keeping me from being the force of change I badly wanted to be.

More and more, I found myself loosening up around my clinical approach. At this time, I also shared the progress I was making with Dr. Sekai Nhiwatiwa, who was a senior psychiatrist and my mentor. She enthusiastically suggested that I stay focused on this important work, as everything we were doing with the Friendship Bench presented possible solutions to the mental healthcare gap that Zimbabweans had faced for too many decades.

Of course, I had selfish reasons for continuing with the work, despite the fact that we had no institutional support to speak of. I enjoyed talking with the grandmothers and learning about their distinctive approach, and the work gave me a sense of purpose that helped assuage the vulnerability and remorse I continued to feel around Erica's death.

Aside from the fact that the Friendship Bench was serving an indirectly therapeutic purpose for me, the message was clear: the community itself could address many of the challenges that mental health professionals had assumed for so many years. Not every problem that the people faced required a specialist or professional who would poke and prod at their "pathologies" through an "objective" lens. People could talk to an empathetic layperson — a loving grandmother — and receive the care they'd probably been in search of all along.

My eyes were wide open, and they stayed that way. All of this experience transformed how I myself provided care to my own patients. I began to emphasize community resources even more than before. And when I interacted with a client at the hospital, I found out who at home or in their community might be able to provide consistent support. If possible, when I connected with someone who lived in Mbare or close by, I thought to link them up with one of the grandmothers or to an existing peer support group. I could imagine that the grand-mothers' bedside manner would help to ease the nerves of many a traumatized or disturbed person who walked through the doors of the hospital, just as it had with Resistance.

Perhaps most notably, I became much more cautious about prescribing medication. It isn't that I believed it wasn't essential; there were certainly situations in which it clearly was. At the same time, context was important. I realized it was premature to put someone on a regimen of medication without knowing more about their story, their struggles, how they'd come to sit before me in the first place. I certainly didn't think it was necessary to put people on antipsychotic medi-cation for lengthy periods of time, which had happened with Resistance. Little by little, just as I was transforming, so was my practice.

I would scarcely have thought it possible, but my discussions with the grandmothers, who seemed to be able to effortlessly contextualize the cognitive behavioral therapy model into a more culturally nuanced and appropriate way of working with people and of seeing the world itself, changed me. Specifically, when it came to facing traditional spiritual and religious beliefs in the community, which sometimes carried their fair share of superstitions and prejudices, the grandmothers were respectful but also encouraged critical thinking and positive action. Above all, they developed a culturally rooted system to navigate through the emotional and psychological issues they were presented with. They understood very well the link between thoughts, feelings, mood, and behavior and how a resulting vicious cycle could lead a client to feeling helpless. They also understood that breaking this cycle at the behavior level through activity scheduling (such as allocating time to communicate with loved ones) and rewarding-behavior activation (like engaging in a collective community action such as making shopping bags that would be sold at the local market) ultimately would lead to a shift in the client's thoughts and feelings. While they were never trained to be professional CBT therapists, they inherently grasped the fundamental connection between positive activity and improved mental well-being.

One afternoon, Grandmother Nhengo shared a story about an HIV-positive man who had been referred by a nurse at his primary healthcare facility. "He was certain he had been bewitched by his late wife, who died after a serious bout of tuberculosis," she recounted. "I listened to his story. He shared a number of challenges he was facing that included being unemployed, struggling to pay his rent, and stigma around his physical symptoms. He joined a group, which has really helped him. In that group, some members have even started income-generation projects as part of their activities."

The income-generation projects that many of the peer

groups had embarked upon were part of the grandmothers' third pillar of care delivery: kusimbisa, or strengthening. When the members of a group worked together, collective cohesion emerged from the team effort and their capacity to problem solve and come to a shared outcome. Many of the groups realized that they could engage in activities that would enable them to make money without any special skills. In fact, a specific grandmother — my own maternal grandmother, who also lived in Mbare — had offered an ingenious idea for how to do this.

I was visiting my eighty-six-year-old grandmother in 2007 when I shared my concerns with her about the community's mental health challenges. "There are so many people struggling with depression, and we've been wanting to bring them together in a meaningful way," I told her. "We know that helping them to realize they have the power to change their circumstances is important. So many of them feel demoralized by poverty, and we want to find ways to help them rise out of this pain together — maybe through some kind of meaningful activity."

My grandmother listened and nodded. I knew I could also receive wise counsel from her, as she was the kind of person who was always happy to lend an ear and tangible advice. She had managed to take care of eight children with very little to her name, except for a piece of land that had become the agricultural patch for the family to grow vegetables seasonally: maize that was consumed and also sold to the community.

Scratching her chin thoughtfully, she said, "Have you thought of using discarded plastic bags and wastepaper?" She sounded proud of her idea and quite certain that it would work, but I didn't understand what she was suggesting.

"What do you mean?"

She leaned in and grinned, as if she were sharing an important secret. "You can make money from most things," she said with a wink, "if you just open your eyes to the opportunity." She showed me how she used a ball of plastic thread to begin crocheting a discarded plastic shopping bag, turning it into a colorful mat. I was stunned. It was such a simple idea, yet it could change the lives of the people being served by the Friendship Bench. It also perfectly dovetailed with the grandmothers' approach, as they had always talked about the need to address the social determinants of kufungisisa in the community — factors like poverty and a sense of purposelessness.

As I watched my grandmother's fingers deftly moving, I couldn't help but think of a favorite phrase of Grandmother Kunehenga, one of the most thoughtful and methodical of all the grandmothers, especially when she spoke up (which wasn't often, compared to the others): "You can't teach a young man how to hunt without a spear."

This idea launched a string of income-creating projects among the existing peer groups. Some of them made a modest community garden where they grew vegetables from organic materials. Another popular project was bread making: each member of the peer group would donate fifty cents toward buying flour, from which they would make the bread to sell. These were simple ideas, but they worked well when it came to generating consistent profit. Not only that, but these activities encouraged sustainability and a direct engagement with the environment and the people of Mbare.

This was part of the glue that was keeping the peer groups together. And it was working…very well.

I learned early on, especially in the midst of our debriefing sessions (which could often be as entertaining as they were enlightening), that the heart of the grandmothers' work was the power of storytelling. They firmly believed that every single one of us has a story to tell — and that even the most heartbreaking story carries within it the possibility of redemption and reconnection to our true nature.

They didn't use exactly those words, but I could see from the way their clients were impacted that they were opening not only community members' minds but also their hearts. I saw more and more people who were eager to step in and offer help, to alleviate the burden of a friend or neighbor in need.

The thing that became very conspicuous to me was the deep level of trust that had been cultivated within these groups. Often, I witnessed participants sacrifice what little they had for the greater good of the group. I had always been skeptical of moneylending schemes, which were common in these circles of community members. I thought they were a surefire way of creating tension and disagreement, but I quickly saw that they provided powerful savings opportunities for the collective. I noticed that when a member needed assistance — perhaps money for a lifesaving operation or for school fees — the others would immediately come together to pool funds for their brother or sister in need, with no concern over whether the money would ever be returned.

I began to realize that people gravitated to the groups because they offer a strong sense of belonging. And with this sense of belonging, opportunities to work together and help one another expand. To that end, even though income generation was one of the initial primary aims of the groups, money isn't the most important glue binding the groups together.

Some of these groups have now been running for a decade or more — and hundreds of new groups continue to form, year after year. Friendship Bench uses a very simple model called asset-based community development (ABCD). It works like this: First, the group establishes the resources (including gifts and talents) that each member can offer. Then, together, they come to a consensus on how they will best utilize these resources. This framework is in stark contrast to some of the well-meaning yet narrow philanthropic models that apply a sort of savior mentality to communities "in need." The savior mentality sees only the deficits of the community and not the collective wealth that might come from a range of different skills. When we are able to recognize the riches that each of us has to contribute, it's as if we activate the skills that everyone brings to the table. People quickly realize, *I have something important to give*, and then they give it.

When the groups began, I believe the grandmothers were revealing to everyone around them the vastness of our human nature; perhaps we are born into unfortunate circumstances, especially those of us struggling with the long aftereffects of intergenerational trauma, but we have a certain amount of power regarding how we respond to such circumstances. And while many people in Mbare had been traumatized by Murambatsvina and a legacy of colonialism and poverty, the grandmothers empowered them to recognize that they had the capacity to move through their trauma with courage and resilience — but first, they needed to feel their feelings and share their stories.

Grandmother Hwiza would often say, "My story of how I lost my teeth and how I spent days being tortured reveals my vulnerability — which is also a strength."

I reflected on this a lot in the first two years of the Friendship Bench. In my career, I had rarely thought of my vulnerability as a strength. When Erica's mother, Sekai, had witnessed my breakdown, I'd felt exposed and somewhat humiliated. The good doctor who was supposed to be providing reassurance needed it himself.

But I could see how much I had softened in the face of the example set by the grandmothers. My reservations had given way to something more profound: the possibility of letting go of the shame-filled emotions I'd locked deep within. Perhaps I could finally forgive myself for Erica's death. Perhaps I could actually accept that I was worthy of forgiveness. Perhaps I could be free.

After one of our regular debriefings, I finally opened up to the grandmothers about my guilt and remorse around Erica's death, which had occurred more than two years earlier. "A patient of mine took her own life, and I haven't been able to let it go," I admitted to them, my voice quavering.

The grandmothers were silent as they listened to me speak. All the details came tumbling out. Perhaps they were surprised, given that I'd been rather tight-lipped about my own problems. After all, so many people in Mbare, including the grandmothers themselves, had dealt with horrific challenges that I felt insulated from. I didn't want to burden other people with my story, and for years I'd believed I had to maintain a clinical distance from the people I worked with, especially my mentees and clients. But the candor of these grandmothers — who routinely shared everything from raucous laughter at crass jokes to the kind of common sense and astuteness only a person with decades of hard-earned life experience could offer — made me realize something: my story mattered, too — and talking about my grief was essential to releasing it.

I hadn't planned any of it, but maybe my "confession" had to be spontaneous in order for it to be authentic. Some part of me still worried that the grandmothers would judge me or think less of me, but with Grandmother Jack's gentle encouragement of "Tell us more," I shared everything. Every memory of Erica: her smile, her constant inquiries about Resistance, her stories of the happiness she'd felt in the mango tree, the way she'd filled the room with her gentleness, how her sadness had seemed to be receding and giving way to hope…until I learned the news of her suicide.

Just as the tears had flowed when I spoke with Sekai for the first time after her daughter's death, they cascaded down my face now. And it wasn't just because I was sharing the story in great detail, but because I felt the warmth and acceptance of fourteen kind pairs of eyes focused on me. I felt their compassion and their healing strength, almost as if I were the baby being rocked to sleep by the voodoo priestess I'd encountered in Benin. I only wished I'd thought to talk to them about Erica much sooner!

At some point in my story, Grandmother Hwiza broke into a soothing, slow, and mellow song. I don't remember the words, but they scarcely mattered. It was a comforting lullaby about being protected in the face of doubt and knowing one's innate strength, despite the presence of painful challenges.

The other thirteen grandmothers joined in to create a calming harmony: Grandmother Chizhande took a deep, low baritone, Grandmother Chinhoyi sang tenor, and Grandmother Kusi assumed alto. I was close to tears once more. Each of the grandmothers instinctively knew where she belonged as she joined the song. But none of it was "performed," none of it orchestrated. They were spontaneously responding to the need for comfort where they saw it. As I listened with the wonderment of a child, I thought of the way my family used to sing together every evening before we went to sleep. Those days seemed relegated to a former time so long ago, but they arose very vividly in my memory as I basked in the grandmothers' melody.

When the song was finished, Grandmother Kusi prayed for me — the same way my mother would pray for me each time I went off on a long journey. That morning, for the first time, I left our debriefing meeting feeling I could heal from Erica's suicide.

It was remarkable. They had not spoken a word. All they had done was sing and pray for me. The sense of relief was astounding. Even after all my epiphanies about the efficacy of their approach, I was left with something I hadn't expected: the embodied experience of feeling totally and unconditionally loved.

In April 2009, just after the seasonal rains stopped, my time with the Friendship Bench underwent another dramatic rite of passage.

Grandmother Jack had attended to more than six hundred clients on the Friendship Bench since we'd started, but this morning was different. She hadn't shown up at all, which was very unlike her. It was after 11 a.m. when Nurse Shelly decided to find out why Grandmother Jack was missing. When she arrived at Grandmother Jack's house, as she would relate to me later that day, she was alarmed to see that a crowd had gathered. A Catholic church choir from the area was singing a mournful song as a group of elderly women chatted in a corner, covering themselves with traditional African clothing — the kind you might see at a funeral.

The day I had known would eventually come and had dreaded had finally transpired. Grandmother Jack was the first of the fourteen grandmothers to pass away. She had died peacefully in her sleep, and her community was saying goodbye as she left for hopefully greener pastures.

People came from all over Mbare to pay their respects to this spitfire of a woman and to bid her farewell. It was bittersweet; on the one hand, it was a clear indication that Grandmother Jack had been deeply revered and appreciated, and on the other, she was leaving at a time when the Friendship Bench most needed her; it was at a major turning point and would likely be expanding demonstrably in a matter of months.

Five days after her death, Resistance was readmitted to the psychiatric hospital. It may have been a coincidence, but given that he and Grandmother Jack had developed a close relationship and she'd continued to support him through his challenges with his community, I felt it was more likely an indication of his own grief and his way of dealing with it. Over time, I'd witnessed Resistance gain greater confidence and clarity, and I knew this was in no small part due to Grandmother Jack's no-nonsense attitude and tough love. For a moment, I worried about what he would do without her support.

There is a popular African proverb: "The death of an elder is equivalent to the burning of a library." While I had intentionally attempted to document most of my interactions with the grandmothers to the best of my ability, as some part of me understood that these stories would serve to inspire others in the future, I recognized in the writing of this book that it was very difficult to do justice to Grandmother Jack.

What could I possibly say about this spirited, strong-willed woman that would adequately describe her powerful legacy? In retrospect, I wish I'd spent more time with her, particularly in the formative months of the Friendship Bench. Today, I am embarrassed to admit that I would deliberately avoid her, as I was annoyed by her eagerness to share her opinions — even though she was often right. Grandmother Jack had challenged all my proclivities and sensibilities as a clinician, but she'd also held the keys to the entire society that I had sought to help. During her funeral, she received many tributes from people; in fact, the service took three hours because of the number of testimonials that people shared about all the good she had done. Even when Zimbabwe had been Rhodesia and Grandmother Jack was just a young girl, she had used her knowledge, wit, sharp tongue, and strong heart in service of others.

I could see that the other grandmothers were heartbroken about this loss. They were almost like a sisterhood, meaning that they bickered about everything but could often find a sense of common ground. Although their candor could sometimes lead to arguments (especially when it came to things like what should have been done or said with respect to a client), they were a team. And, as I've learned over the years, nothing creates a sense of cohesion and closeness among the grandmothers quite as much as the death of one of their own.

I knew that the Friendship Bench, which had benefited greatly from Grandmother Jack's generosity, would continue to flourish because of the love she'd poured into it — and I also knew it would not be the same without her. As with many powerful pillars of their community, this beautiful matriarch's time with us had been much too brief.

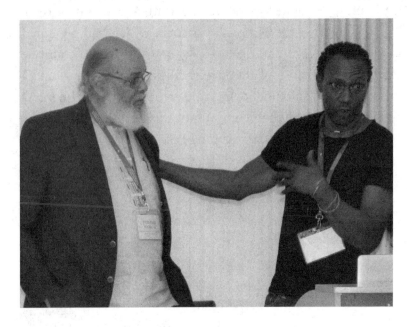

Introducing Fred Hickling to PhD students from the African Mental Health Research Initiative (AMARI) in Lilongwe, Malawi.

Chapter Seven

Fred

I always knew that the grandmothers would eventually leave this plane of existence. After all, despite their vim and vigor, they were also elderly and frail. However, some naive part of me never really faced the reality that I would lose them...that is, until Grandmother Jack's death. It was a sad realization. I felt a sense of anguish and loss, as well as desperation. Which of the grandmothers would be the next to go? To this day, every time one of the original grandmothers dies, it leaves an emptiness inside me that cannot be filled. I still haven't grown accustomed to it.

With the awareness that our time together was limited, I was driven to establish even closer bonds with the grandmothers who remained. Grandmother Jack's death opened my eyes to the inevitability of loss and the impermanence of everything around us, of life in general. Trying to hold on was futile, but at the very least, I could value the precious time we still had. I began to ritualize our celebrations with more regularity. Having Christmas meetings with the grandmothers — during which we would feast, share stories, pray, and sing together — became something I looked forward to every year.

After Grandmother Jack's death, we began to ask in earnest how we could leverage the lessons that the grandmothers had acquired, so that we could ensure their legacy would spread far and wide. We had many well-wishers, as well as a modest grant from a UK-based charitable organization, Zimbabwe Health Training Support, which came in the wake of our first peer-reviewed publication in 2009.

The grant enabled us to buy mobile phones for the grandmothers, as well as shoes and Friendship Bench–branded T-shirts, but it was time to think through our own income-generating ideas for ways to keep our enterprise afloat. In the three years we'd been serving the communities of Harare, most of the expenses for the Friendship Bench had continued to be paid out of my pocket. It was costing me the equivalent of $100 USD a month to support the grandmothers with stationery and a small communication allowance. I was dreading the moment when I would be unable to support any further activity…and I knew that moment was going to be coming very soon.

The first peer-reviewed paper published about the Friendship Bench examined the effects of group therapy on postnatal depression and how the peer support groups that emerged from the Friendship Bench helped mothers struggling with this issue. The paper was inspired by the mentor I mentioned earlier, Dr. Sekai Nhiwatiwa, the head of psychiatry at the University of Zimbabwe, who had continued to stress the importance of creating an evidence-based foundation for the work I was doing with the grandmothers. Even though this was of very little importance to the grandmothers, who were more interested in being of service than in gathering proof that their method was working, all of us knew what was needed if we wanted our endeavors to receive support, especially in the way of exposure that would lead to funding.

The peer-reviewed paper also opened the way for further collaboration with UK partners, who would publish a more extensive pilot study that demonstrated the efficacy of the grandmothers' approach for treating depression in a low-resource, low-income setting.

After that first peer-reviewed publication, the floodgates opened, and the Friendship Bench received an influx of international attention. In 2010, Grand Challenges Canada (GCC) approached us and encouraged me to apply for a larger grant. They were a brand-new nonprofit organization that funded solutions to critical health challenges in the developing world. They'd eventually go on to fund more than a thousand projects in close to one hundred countries around the world, but at this stage, they were just getting started. Peter Singer, the CEO of Grand Challenges Canada, was keen to support the Friendship Bench, even though we were still very much a one-man and now thirteen-grandmother show.

The first grant we received from the organization was roughly $800,000 USD, and it supported the first clinical trial I ever administered. It was a huge process, meant to evaluate the effectiveness of the Friendship Bench on overall health outcomes in Mbare. A clinical trial goes through multiple phases: pretrial preparation, followup, data analysis, and submission for publication. Ours took more than two years, and in that time, some of the funding was allocated toward an initial training during which the thirteen remaining grandmothers educated even more grandmothers across Harare, who would also participate in the clinical trial. The concluding analysis was published in the *Journal of the American*

Medical Association — no small feat for what had started as a grassroots initiative that I'd bootstrapped from scarce resources and a broken heart.

When we were still in the process of analyzing the results of the clinical trial, all of the individuals and organizations from GCC's initial cohort of grantees were invited to present their preliminary findings in Toronto. And so it was during the fall of 2012 that I arrived in Toronto, eager to share the work of the Friendship Bench at the first meeting of cohorts.

As I disembarked from the airplane, my initial excitement was dampened by a phenomenon that far too many people of color are familiar with: traveling while Black. I was singled out for what the security officer casually described as a routine random check. The initial pleasantries, however, quickly gave way to something that felt more sinister. The officer was a blond woman in her mid-thirties.

"Where are you flying from, sir?" she asked.

"Africa."

"With just hand luggage?"

"Yes. I always travel with just hand luggage."

"Why, sir?"

I smiled, somewhat amused by the obvious question. "Because it makes life easier."

"Sir, we need to search your bag," she demanded, her voice suddenly more serious and authoritative. I obliged.

She took my bag and ran a white swab around the interior and exterior. She walked up to a machine and carefully placed the swab inside, as if she were collecting medical evidence at the scene of a crime. After a few minutes, she walked back to me. "Sir, have you ever taken cocaine in your life?" she asked.

"No." *Where is this all coming from?* I wondered.

"Sir, do you have cocaine in your bag?"

I was firm — and stern. "No. I have no cocaine anywhere in my bag or on my person."

"We'll have to search your entire bag, then," she said, as if she were looking forward to proving me wrong.

"Sure, please go ahead." I was curious as to what she'd say when she came up empty-handed.

My personal belongings were strewn unceremoniously across a table as the security officer sifted through each item thoroughly and with great interest. "Why do you have all these tablets in your toilet bag?" she inquired, spilling its contents onto the table.

"That's loperamide." I pointed at the little capsules. "It's for diarrhea. It stops you —"

She put up a hand and gave me a disgusted look. "You don't have to go into the details," she said, cutting me off. "And this?"

"Paracetamol. And that's Brufen, which is an anti-inflammatory. That's amoxicillin, which is an antibiotic. And that's —"

She frowned as she cut me off once more. "Why do you have to carry all these tablets? Are you a doctor?"

I responded, "Yes, I'm a doctor." She seemed surprised.

I thought that perhaps this would be the end of it, as I clearly had no illegal substances on me. But I was wrong. I spent more than an hour being interrogated by the security officer, who seemed hell-bent on getting me to admit that I had cocaine. Certainly, I understood that the smuggling of illegal drugs was a security risk in any nation, but I was at a loss as to why I had been detained when it was clear that I was a doctor on his way to an international convening of people who were doing innovative, socially responsible work in their respective countries. But nothing I said seemed to matter. She had apparently made up her mind: in her eyes, even if there was no cocaine to be found in my possession, I was guilty of *something*.

Assisted by a stony-eyed young man who looked like he'd just come out of college, the security officer removed every article of clothing in my hand luggage *and* made me strip down until I was almost naked. I was also forced to give them my laptop password; I watched in angry silence as they scanned through my documents. Finally, an older, bearded White man arrived, and the two walked away to chat with him privately as I stood awkwardly in a small security cubicle.

The security officer came back. "You can go," she said abruptly, offering nothing in the way of an apology or even an explanation.

I was humiliated, but I understood this was probably par for the course.

Welcome to Canada.

The scheduled bus to the hotel had already left by the time I cleared immigration. I opted for a cab and silently licked my emotional wounds as I headed to the hotel.

I was standing in front of the hotel reception counter behind four guests waiting to be checked in. What should have been a celebratory occasion — sharing the initial findings of a clinical trial that had been several years in the making — had been deflated by the airport incident. Most of me was wishing I hadn't set foot in this godforsaken country.

I waited quietly, marinating in the anger and disbelief of what had been such a rude and disparaging welcome. *So much for hospitality!*

Suddenly, my thoughts were interrupted by a voice. "You look troubled, my brother." The voice had a distinct Caribbean accent.

When I looked up, I saw a tall, bearded Black man gazing down at me with kindly eyes.

"I've had the most miserable day of my life," I admitted, so angry and dejected that I didn't think of sparing this stranger the details. "As soon as I arrived at the airport, I was selected for a random search."

He smiled sympathetically. "How many Black people were on the plane?" His deep Jamaican accent reminded me of Azagba, my enthusiastic tour guide in Benin.

"I was the only one," I said, wondering why that hadn't occurred to me at the time.

"And it sounds like this was the first time you were subjected to this kind of treatment. Well, let me tell you something, my brother." He got closer and reassuringly placed one massive hand on my shoulder. "It won't be the last time. My name is Fred." He stroked his white Santa beard thoughtfully. "There are some basic rules you need to know about traveling while Black. Why don't you finish your check-in and then let's meet in the lobby?"

This would be my first encounter with Dr. Fred Hickling, but certainly not my last.

Fred was one of GCC's grantees, a psychiatrist from Jamaica who had set up his organization, the Caribbean Institute of Mental Health and Substance Abuse (CARIMENSA), after observing the troubles of disadvantaged young people across the island nation. Unsurprisingly, we became fast friends. We would come to find out that we shared a great deal of common ground. Like me, Fred had discovered the importance of working to empower people within the community to take their mental health into their own hands. He had come to the conclusion that many instances of psychotic episodes could be managed within the community, with enough care and education. Most of the people he worked with were volunteers, but he also engaged a number of psychiatrists and nurses who provided guidance and support.

While the Friendship Bench dealt primarily with depression, anxiety, and PTSD, Fred and his team were focused mostly on addressing substance abuse and also on providing a safe and empowering space for young people who had been labeled by the authorities as troublemakers caught in a seemingly inescapable maze of gang violence and a general sense of aimlessness. Both Fred and I were invested in doing what we could to help people caught in a cycle of poverty and trauma to see themselves in a new light. But now, Fred was also making me aware of the fact that I would have to face doubt and disparagement from people who questioned my authority, and even my right to be in certain spaces, as a Black man. He would challenge me to see myself in a new light as well.

Every single one of us could benefit from a wise older friend who's seen and done it all — someone with whom we can sit down and have a cup of tea and release all our frailties, fears, and vulnerabilities without the fear of being judged. Fred quickly became that person for me.

In many ways, Fred served a similar purpose in my life as the grandmothers. The grandmothers and Fred were rooted in their respective communities and were intimately connected to the stories of people on the ground. However, unlike the grandmothers, who were not well-off by any means, Fred came from a fairly wealthy family in Jamaica. At the same time, they all shared the mentality that culture was a potent form of therapy, one that could instill a sense of pride and meaning in people who felt unmoored and bereft of opportunity. Obviously, Fred had the added advantage of being an educated psychiatrist with a global understanding of the world, but it was his gift of being able to immerse himself in the lives and struggles of the people he helped that stood out to me and made me recognize him as a kindred spirit.

Fred told me that he'd started his career in the United Kingdom. During his stint there, he noticed that people of color — particularly those of Black and Asian origin — were more likely than White people to be involuntarily admitted into psychiatric hospitals for psychotic illness. This inspired Fred to begin investigating the root causes behind the discrepancy.

During that period, he wrote a book called *Owning Our Madness*. The major thesis of the book was that true healing cannot happen until Black and Asian people go back to their cultural roots, where they may come to understand some of the major expressions of stress within that culture rather than relying on Western definitions of "madness." One of the foundations of Fred's work was the importance of people of color rooting back into their Indigenous communities, which he saw as a radical act of reclamation and restitution. As Fred began to work more deeply with people in Jamaica, he dug into the lingering effects of the slave trade, as well as the role of generational violence. Much of his work was around understanding how communities perceive healing. In a way, he was also removing himself from existing frameworks, something I was striving to do. Because Fred had been engaged in this work for a long time, it gave me hope.

After the Toronto conference, Fred and I established a channel of regular communication that was grounded in genuine empathy. Fred had devoted himself to learning about local culture and Indigenous wisdom, as well as cultural idioms of distress, long before I had even considered the therapeutic value of these things. For years, CARIMENSA had offered a wide range of outreach services, developing culturally appropriate interventions in which community wisdom and creativity were used to explore and express painful issues.

One of Fred's initiatives, which was also being supported by GCC, was the award-winning Dream-a-World Cultural Therapy project, which focused on inner-city communities plagued with gang violence and high rates of teenage pregnancies. In a scientifically elegant and structured way, Fred and his team had emphasized the importance of what my grandmothers in Mbare were articulating as critical factors in addressing mental health. He'd coined the term *psychohistoriography*, which he defined as the creative exploration of social, personal, and cultural issues as therapeutic treatment. I enjoyed sharing about my debriefing sessions with the grandmothers with Fred, who often responded with, "Your grandmothers are an important source of oral tradition and history — learn from them!"

In private conversations, Fred encouraged me to be aware of the effects of internalized racism, a term that was new to me when he mentioned it at our first meeting. In the same spirit of the grandmothers, especially Grandmother Jack, Fred would send me on my way with book recommendations in the hope that they would open up my mind to an issue I hadn't even considered.

Internalized racism is defined by the Black American physician and epidemiologist Camara Phyllis Jones as "a stigmatized race's internalization and acceptance of external negative messages about their abilities and intrinsic worth." It involves accepting perceived limitations to one's full humanity, which encompasses dreams, self-determination, and the range of allowable self-expression. For example, I came to understand there is an unspoken edict that Black people should not express anything that approaches anger, for fear of being branded as "the angry Black person."

I realized that cold evening in Toronto when I first met Fred and he talked to me about internalized racism that I had been a victim of it through my own failure to sufficiently respond to the inhumane treatment I had received from the airport security officers.

"Like most people of color out there, you conveniently played the part," Fred said, with a firmness that managed to be kind.

Although I sensed the wisdom in his words, my immediate knee-jerk reaction was resistance. I was uncomfortable with what he was suggesting to me, but this changed over time as he gradually shared his own stories.

"Jamaica has a rich culture, but the scars of colonialism are so deep that people still want to emulate Western standards and ways of seeing the world," he told me. Fred had navigated the global mental health sphere long enough to map the co-ordinates. But, as he divulged, his journey of untangling the threads of internalized racism, especially as a young psychiatrist who sought to emulate the White medical establishment, had been anything but easy.

While we continued to see each other at meetings around the world, especially as the Friendship Bench project eventually grew beyond Harare, most of our conversations took place via WhatsApp. Fred had a knack for asking me simple questions that turned into complex, soulful conversations; often, they had little or nothing to do with the academic content of my work, but were much more centered around how I was navigating my role as a leader of a growing organization.

"What's been the most difficult thing for you at a personal level?" he asked me one day.

As I opened up to Fred, I shared my struggles with relating to people (one in particular) who didn't respect my position as the director of the Friendship Bench initiative. This person was a digital expert who was dismissive of the work I was doing with the grandmothers from the outset. Surprisingly, he sounded like a clinician whenever he shared his unsolicited opinion that I should be leaving this work to "professionals." I eventually asked him to leave the growing organization, which resulted in an unfortunate legal skirmish. In the end, he did go, but it was a difficult situation all the same — especially because I still had many residual doubts about the effectiveness and value of what we were doing.

It was Fred who bolstered my spirits and helped me to remain resolute in the face of setbacks. He continued to re-assure me that the Friendship Bench model was coming up against opposition only because it was so novel. Since it was not rooted in a traditional psychiatric framework, naturally people would be reluctant to recognize the legitimacy of our work. Thanks to Fred, I felt supported in doing everything I could to keep going, even when I wanted to do exactly the opposite.

The more we discussed the matter over the years, the more I recognized that the topic of our very first conversation was still pertinent. Despite my Western education and my own passion for dispelling stereotypes about Africa and her people, I still hadn't fully come to terms with the extent of my internalized racism.

Fred was helpful as I worked my way to these growing, and excruciatingly difficult, realizations. "You need to know what is right, but you also need to choose your battles carefully," he said, "because as a Black person, if you choose to be angry all the time, you'll be fighting battles every single day of your life — and then everything will feel meaningless."

Fred's challenge to me was clear: "How are you going to help those coming behind you to address their internalized racism? Young people working with you will look to you as a mentor, and the choices you make now will be important — not just for you, but also for them." I had no response to his question at the time, although it would stay with me for years and inspire more realizations and possibilities, just as the guilt around Erica's suicide had planted the seed for the Friendship Bench.

As the Friendship Bench project grew, Fred remained an important friend, ally, and colleague. Predictably, he managed to rankle a number of my White collaborating research partners, who were uncomfortable with the intensity of his rhetoric. He was the first academic of color I had met who would gladly take the bull by the horns by publicly acknowledging the proverbial elephant in the room: the ugly lingering legacy of colonialism and the slave trade, what it had done to Black people globally, and what it continued to do in professional circles. Those professional circles included the global mental health space, where so many well-meaning professionals managed to skirt around the effects of an entrenched intergenerational trauma that was not so easy to shrug off… and that could not so easily be healed by Western medical interventions.

"Fred Hickling is irritating and racist," a colleague candidly declared to me. "In fact, he's downright toxic!"

It wasn't easy. I was working with a multiracial team, with collaborating partners from the United States, the United Kingdom, and many other places. I felt loyal to Fred, who was undoubtedly a valuable mentor, but I was also learning to diplomatically navigate many different personalities — especially when it came to the minefield of racism, which was a less talked about subject in the 2010s than it is now.

Fred felt I was vulnerable and gullible and that I needed to be firmer and more assertive in my own convictions and practices. Just as the grandmothers had opened my mind to more therapeutic possibilities, Fred did the same in the realm of literature. He introduced me to the work of Frantz Fanon, the French West Indian psychiatrist who'd written books like *The Wretched of the Earth* and become one of the greatest postcolonial voices on the planet. Fred also encouraged me to read the works of literary giants like James Baldwin, Ngugi wa Thiong'o, and Maya Angelou, as well as other important thinkers who weren't interested in merely bucking the system but wanted to transform it from the inside out.

Even when Fred inadvertently placed me between the proverbial rock and a hard place, I admired him immensely. He didn't seem to mind being labeled a racist when I confronted him and said that his strong language was creating a rift with our other collaborators. His response was swift and sure. "White privilege is real. Any White person who truly acknowledges White privilege will strive to use it to level the playing field rather than perpetuate existing inequalities. I advise you to stay away from any White person who does not want to do this."

Privately, he always emphasized that everything he was sharing was not a negation of White people or Western culture; rather, it was about ensuring that people of color had equal opportunities and that we came to grips with the legacy of the slave trade, colonialism, and racism, a legacy that was still very much alive and well.

I recall one cold afternoon in Cape Town, South Africa, when Fred said to me, "The bullet is a means of physical subjugation and language the means for spiritual subjugation." He looked at me intently. "Do you know who said this?"

"No," I replied.

"Ngugi wa Thiong'o. Read his works. Of course, when you state a fact that is painful, you'll be labeled," he went on. "I've asked myself if I want to state facts and live with being labeled or be quiet and be considered a good person. I know what my answer is. Do you?"

Fred's influence on me had huge personal and professional ramifications. When I received funding for the African Mental

Health Research Initiative, a grant administered through Developing Excellence in Leadership, Training, and Science in Africa, I invited Fred to sit on my independent advisory team, along with Vikram Patel, a prominent Harvard University psychiatrist. I thrived with Fred's support, and much of what I went on to achieve with the Friendship Bench I owed to him. Fred had a great deal of experience in building capacity at a local level and in empowering community members to recognize and own their own worth. In our conversations, he often emphasized that too many people of color tended to believe they were not capable of achieving great things, not necessarily because it's what they consciously believed, but because a history of subjugation under colonial rule can create all kinds of unconscious misconceptions.

In a way, Fred and Grandmother Jack served the same purpose in my growth — Fred through an academic lens, Grandmother Jack through a personal wisdom that was rooted in her decades of practical lived experience and had the backing of many generations of oral history and tradition. Despite their differences, they were linked by their shared ability to speak truth to power, to tell it like it is. Both of them were revered elders in my life, helping me to see what I had not previously seen and to navigate my growth edges with some grace…and perhaps even a sense of humor.

But Fred also departed at a time when I desperately needed guidance. Sadly, he passed away in 2021; like Grandmother Jack, he died peacefully in his sleep.

A period of loneliness and despair often follows the loss of personal anchors. Fred was one of my most trusted anchors, and I didn't know if I would ever again come across the same unique combination of friendship, professional camaraderie, and deep wisdom that he had offered me. Fred had turned a most undignified experience — my first encounter with Canada — into a learning opportunity. And, similar to the grandmothers, Fred had impressed upon me the importance of tapping into a source of power that went beyond the approval of my peers: the source of power that inevitably led to becoming an elder who both trusted in the radiance of their own light and had the power to inspire new generations in search of a better path forward.

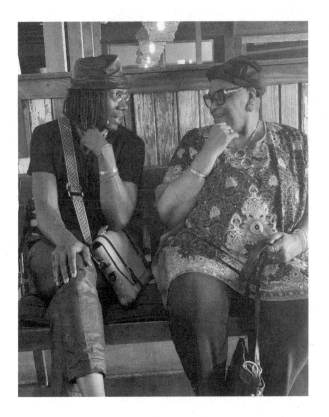

Discussing the Friendship Bench New Orleans project with Carole Bebele in 2023. Almost seven years after my TED Talk, Carole got in touch about starting a Friendship Bench program in New Orleans. She has continued to be an amazing leader on my journey to expand the program.

Chapter Eight

A Connected World

O ur clinical trial on the effectiveness of mental health intervention delivered by lay health workers took place
primarily between 2014 and 2016. Our results, published in
the prestigious *Journal of the American Medical Association* in
2016, created waves around the world and brought many a curious international visitor to Harare. (Following Fred's advice
that "if you have strong evidence, go for the jugular," we aimed
for the highest-impact publication we possibly could.) It was
my first major publication with my name as first author, and I
will always be indebted to the great team from King's College
London, London School of Hygiene and Tropical Medicine,
and the University of Zimbabwe who made it possible, many
of whom I continue to work with.

The results of the trial were startling: six months after receiving therapy from a trained community grandmother,
people who'd had symptoms of depression and anxiety were
symptom-free. In fact, it turned out that the grandmothers
were a lot better at reducing symptoms of common mental disorders than your typical trained professionals were; 80 percent
of people who came to the Friendship Bench had better mental

health outcomes than those who received enhanced care, such as medication or treatment from a licensed clinician.

And thus began a period of exponential growth. Suddenly, the Friendship Bench and the grandmothers had the eyes of the world upon us. Peter Singer, the CEO of Grand Challenges Canada, was especially ecstatic at the findings surfaced by the clinical trial in 2016. Because of his own cultural background and the memory of his beloved Jewish grandmother, who'd played a powerful role in his upbringing, he was eager to see how a community could come together to heal the anguish of its people. That year Peter came to Zimbabwe to experience firsthand the work of the grandmothers.

During this visit, we were in an intensive process of scaling and training the additional grandmothers who were pouring into the project. We were also continuing to recognize the power of the peer support groups. Peter was keen on attending a support group, so I took him to the low-income suburb of Kuwadzana, where I introduced him to the community, as well as the staff of the nearby primary clinical facility that provided care for anyone who required more intensive medical attention. Peter had the chance to interact with both the grandmothers and the clients, absorbing their stories, learning why they'd come to the Friendship Bench to begin with, and hearing about how it had transformed their lives.

Visiting the community with Peter revealed just how much the grandmothers had achieved while also highlighting the support that we still needed to make this intervention available in all communities across Harare. Our goal was to have a Friendship Bench within walking distance of people's homes everywhere in the city. We wanted to ensure that people like Erica would easily have someone to talk to, rather than being forced to make a long trek to a clinic where they might not even receive adequate support to get them through a difficult time.

For more than three years, I had been working exclusively with the grandmothers from Mbare, but on this sunny April morning, against the backdrop of a terra-cotta wall, an army of the next generation of grandmothers proceeded to take their positions as we prepared to start our group meeting. The group gathered in a circle to welcome our international visitor with singing and dancing. This was followed by testimonials from individuals who had received services from the Friendship Bench.

I distinctly remember the brave accounts of people living with HIV who'd found the bench, and particularly the support groups, lifesaving. People in the community, including the grandmothers, had become much more aware of the challenges associated with lack of treatment. In turn, this created a greater sense of collective commitment and responsibility when it came to caring for the people who most needed it.

One of the clients, Marita, had presented with an alarmingly high SSQ score of ten before being invited to receive sessions on the bench, which subsequently led to her joining one of the community support groups. The circle quieted down as we all focused on Marita, who had the talking piece in her hand.

"I still remember the day I tested HIV positive," she said in a voice that was both soft and strong. "I had been struggling with general body malaise and coughing with swelling of lymph nodes in my neck. On top of that, I was pregnant." Tears fell from her eyes. She gestured to the sleeping infant strapped to her back. "This is my child. He is HIV negative because I was put on the prevention of mother-to-child transmission program. I didn't know about this program until I came to the Friendship Bench. I owe so much to the support I received here, to the grandmothers who listened to and helped me, and to the people in the group who also provided me with kindness and care."

I could see that Peter was in awe of the work we were doing. After his visit, he mused about the beautiful simplicity of our approach. He felt that being in a circle with a group of people, where one person was holding the talking piece and was the center of caring attention for as long as they held it, was an extremely potent way of creating space for individuals to share while ensuring that the collective bond was strong enough to provide validation to each person who told their story.

Peter had always been a strong advocate of community, and like both Fred and me, he believed that addressing the social determinants of mental health began and ended within the community. He was also moved by the stories that emerged from the peer support groups: engaging, heartbreaking accounts of intimate partner violence, poverty, and children struggling to find a way to go to school. The human element and the innovative ways in which the groups helped participants to work through adversity captured Peter's heart and imagination, just as they had mine.

He continued to be a champion for us and even to promote our work when he went on to become a senior advisor to the current director of the World Health Organization. Peter also continued to gently direct people to the Friendship Bench, and I'd like to believe he played a major role in drawing attention to the fact that ours was a model that could be easily replicated and used in various parts of the world.

In fact, the Friendship Bench became part of a massive special initiative from WHO that focused on strengthening mental health in seven countries; this led to our organization working closely with both WHO and the national government of Zimbabwe. Although Peter wasn't directly involved, his advocacy had helped launch us onto the global stage in ways that I would never have been able to imagine a few years earlier.

All the difficulties I'd encountered, from my incessant self-doubt to my run-ins with people who didn't respect my authority, ended up paying off. With the assistance of the grants we received from GCC, we were able to provide Friendship Bench with peer-education trainings to cover the remainder of Harare's communities in 2014 and 2015. It was the culmination of a dream we'd had for years, one that at the outset we weren't certain was achievable.

The grandmothers who'd been with us from the beginning assisted our training team to carry out trainings in three batches over several months — as peer supervisors this time around. By the end of this period, we had approximately eighty grandmothers providing support and opening the minds of people all over Harare, while the original Mbare grandmothers were the revered elders who held it all together with a newfound sense of authority. I was delighted to see that all of them were conspicuously elevated in the eyes of the grandmothers they were training. And although she was not part of the trainings, the late Grandmother Jack's singular stamp was all over the work we were doing.

It was a new era for the Friendship Bench. Although we continued to lose some of the original grandmothers, we remained determined and industrious. Throughout the mourning of our revered elders — the original grandmothers whose time with us had come and gone — we managed to ensure that the patients with the greatest needs were each assigned a grandmother who would help tether them back to their lives and communities. Resistance, for example, who was initially heartbroken after Grandmother Jack's death, was comforted by the kindness of Grandmother Kandawasvika, who lived close to him and was the perfect person to step into Grandmother Jack's shoes to offer solace and support.

It all clicked into place one day when I talked to Resistance and saw the light in his eyes as he spoke of his conversations with the grandmothers. I understood that they had given him a sense of purpose and community. He felt recognized as a human being. Simply waking up and knowing that he would be having a conversation with a grandmother later that day bolstered his hope. A simple connection enabled Resistance to thrive in unforeseen ways. Such a small thing made such a big difference — and this is typically true for most of us.

By now, we'd also accumulated a significant number of peer-reviewed scientific publications to validate the claims we were making. Our primary message was that ordinary people could contribute to narrowing the worrisome mental health-care gap. As the custodians of the local culture and wisdom, grandmothers in particular had a pivotal role to play. They were familiar with the struggles of the people around them, and the respect they commanded enabled them to destigmatize any lingering concerns around mental health issues.

One of the things that made me proudest of the work we

were doing was the respect that was being given to the grand-mothers. Frankly, I felt it was long overdue. While I was the face of the Friendship Bench, at least in an international sense and when it came to fielding questions from mental health professionals around the world, a number of international media outlets, from the BBC to CNN, had come to recognize the extraordinary work of the grandmothers.

The most compelling human interest stories, in fact, were the ones that featured the grandmothers in their "natural hab-itat" — offering solace to the people who came to see them. They shared their homegrown wisdom with human beings who were hungry for the kind of love only a grandmother could give, for the compassionate reflection that would help them to know they were not broken and that, in fact, a way ex-isted out of their pain and suffering. In retrospect, I wondered if Erica would have benefited from such a sensibility — a no-nonsense approach saturated with deep compassion and the sort of valuable, freely offered life lessons one wouldn't necessarily receive from a mental health professional alone.

I was especially proud that the original grandmothers were able to bask in the limelight and receive so much rec-ognition for their years of hard work. By now, they'd proven to be the gold standard in how a Friendship Bench could and should operate. The grandmothers from Harare's other com-munities often came to visit the ones in Mbare to see how they were faring and to bring them gifts in recognition of their important work; it almost seemed like a sort of pilgrimage to the epicenter and heart of the project, where the passion and laughter were as strong as ever.

Given that so many elders, especially women, do not re-ceive the recognition and appreciation they rightfully deserve,

I have always felt that the Friendship Bench offers a beautiful reciprocity that honors the place of the archetypal grandmother in our society.

I once visited Grandmother Kusi at her home, and it was gratifying to see how generations of family members, all the way down to the grandchildren, were proud of her and grateful that she was being recognized on an international level. I think we all have the innate desire to be needed and to have our unique talents and offerings received wholeheartedly. I knew that this wasn't about the grandmothers feeding their egos; it was about reveling in the awareness that what they had to share mattered and that it had the power to change lives.

They didn't have to be CEOs or PhDs — their hearts and commitment were more than enough to inspire the world. I believe this gave Grandmother Kusi and the others the confidence to fully inhabit the social role they were playing; all of them were often called upon to discuss a variety of community issues in different settings. Aside from being revered within the immediate community of those who came to the Friendship Bench, they were asked to be keynote speakers at conferences and other events. They were finally being recognized as the experts they were — as the ones who had opened the hearts and minds of so many people, including me.

If you were to ask the grandmothers today what continues to inspire them to do the work, they would unanimously say that while it's certainly about helping others, the Friendship Bench has also enabled them to become better, more compassionate, and more socially engaged people.

When Grandmother Chinhoyi was on her deathbed, I sat in a little room where she was lying on a small cot; her breathing was labored, and I could sense that she might leave us at any moment. It was profoundly painful, but I was grateful to be there with her, as I hadn't been able to say goodbye to Grandmother Jack.

I held Grandmother Chinhoyi's small hand in mine, and she looked up at me with a beautiful smile. "I want you to know, Doctor, that being part of the Friendship Bench has given me a sense of purpose and belonging that I don't think I would have otherwise had." We sat there wordlessly, held together in a sacred silence. I could feel that her words were her way of saying goodbye to me.

A few hours after I left, accompanied by Dr. Ruth Verhey, the senior clinical psychologist at the Friendship Bench, I received the news that Grandmother Chinhoyi was gone. It was a bittersweet moment, as it has been every time I've received news that one of the fourteen original grandmothers has passed away — filled with sadness but also appreciation for the gifts that these incredible women have given me.

I had never had the pleasure of being able to sit with any of the other grandmothers prior to their death, as most of them had passed unexpectedly, so there was something about this experience that felt deeply healing to me. I always regretted that I'd not been able to let Grandmother Jack know how much she meant to me, but sitting in that little room with Grandmother Chinhoyi's tiny hand in mine gave me a sense of peace and closure. All that I'd never gotten a chance to say before, I was able to express in just a few minutes, and no words were necessary. I believe that Grandmother Chinhoyi and I felt the enormity and emotional presence of the last several years in our final moments together.

Aside from the dramatic changes that were occurring with respect to the Friendship Bench, I was undergoing a realization of my own. In 2016, I made the decision to resign from my position at the hospital, where I'd been working for close to thirteen years.

Ever since Erica's death and my subsequent work with the grandmothers, I knew that I wanted to transform the hospital into a more supportive therapeutic community — a place that was associated with healing rather than shame and stigma. As I was deepening my own dedication to community mental health, I knew that reforming the clinical setting was vital to the kind of widespread transformation I wanted to see.

I attempted to fundraise around developing a new facility, a patient-centered environment where the people who came to see us would feel comfortable and cared for. Whereas the hospital placed an emphasis on the medicalization of any and all human suffering, I was already aware from my work with the Friendship Bench that the vast majority of the people we treated didn't need medication. Although I knew that suggesting new policies might not be immediately welcomed, I figured that I could at least propose changes to our environment: I recommended that we make it more user-friendly for staff and clients and that we introduce alternative forms of therapy, including martial arts and yoga.

However, the hospital authorities had very different ideas, which they made unambiguously known. It was a shock and a disappointment to realize that transformation of the facility was impossible. I knew then and there that I wouldn't be able to continue my work at the hospital.

I originally thought I'd resign from my position altogether and devote my time to the Friendship Bench, but after Fred heard me out while I shared my grievances, he said, "If you leave the hospital, you should consider teaching at the university. That way, you'll still be able to have a presence at the hospital, where you can continue to support patients in some way. You'll also have some institutional support for continuing your work with the Friendship Bench."

It had never occurred to me that I could maintain a relationship with the hospital by transitioning into an academic setting. I had already been involved with the University of Zimbabwe as an honorary lecturer and had collaborated with UZ on a number of studies linked to the Friendship Bench, so stepping into academia full-time would simply formalize my arrangement. Fred also advised me to apply for a position in London, so I could enjoy a joint role that would enable me to stay connected to the community in Harare while growing my global network and meeting potential new partners in Europe and other parts of the world.

And so, in 2017, I resigned from my job at the hospital and took a position as an associate professor at the University of Zimbabwe. Then, in 2018, I also accepted a position at the London School of Hygiene and Tropical Medicine, where I took Fred's original words and ideas to heart.

I noticed that many of my students from Asia and Africa, bright as they were, tended toward timidity and doubted themselves a great deal. In some ways, despite all they'd already accomplished, they suffered from the same poverty of mind that the grandmothers had discussed with me — a poverty that far transcended their actual circumstances and encompassed the ideas about their deeper self-worth (or lack thereof) that they'd imbibed from their environment.

I was committed to taking my students through a process of undoing their limitations, just as Fred had done with me. My newfound freedom as a professor gave me a cohesive way to bridge my academic work with my Friendship Bench work, and I was even able to integrate my students and their research interests into what I was doing with the grandmothers.

Fred proved to be correct in other ways, too. In the period of time when we started the larger peer-education trainings with the grandmothers, I realized we needed to bring on a project coordinator who would oversee all the logistics. When I had begun my association with the University of Zimbabwe in 2014, the Friendship Bench became nested within the university. In 2017 we broke from that arrangement to form our own autonomous, fully fledged organization. Fred's prescience and stellar advice had once again proven to be valuable.

Now that I was in a university position that gave me more time and freedom to spend on research, I was able to develop even more ideas about how the Friendship Bench could be used to help people in the community. Ironically, while I had failed to establish a therapeutic community inside the hospital, I would eventually do so when the Friendship Bench became a self-supporting organization.

In 2018, we created the first Friendship Bench Hub, a beautiful facility in Harare that was designed with a therapeutic effect in mind. At the Friendship Bench Hub, we offered free therapy, as well as other restorative practices. We even had a swimming pool and benches in the garden, where visitors could sit and talk with trained peer counselors or a grandmother if one was available. The previous limitations I'd encountered in the hospital setting were no longer an impediment to my work. I was heartened by the fact that even though I hadn't been able to make the difference I'd wanted to at the hospital, everything I'd intended to do was coming to fruition — and in more far-reaching ways.

In 2017, the same year that the Friendship Bench finally became a formally autonomous organization, I found myself traveling to New Orleans and giving a talk on the main stage of TED Talks.

It had all started in Aspen, Colorado. I was a fellow with the Aspen Global Innovators New Voices Fellowship, which trained experts and advocates from countries across the world to employ communications, advocacy, and storytelling in ways that would shift public opinion and policy. During that meeting in Aspen, I spoke about the Friendship Bench in five minutes, and people immediately took notice. There was such an interest, in fact, that a wealthy couple I met that day invited me to their place for dinner. They lived in a massive house on the river, and they offered me a cigar to smoke. Little did I know that one doesn't inhale while smoking a cigar; my lack of experience caused me to nearly choke! I was a fish out of water in more ways than one.

During that trip, I was also approached by media pioneer Pat Mitchell, who was now the director of TEDWomen. "You need to tell your story on a bigger stage — the world should hear it!" she exclaimed. Prior to this, I hadn't even heard about TED. Not long afterward, I received an email from the organizers of TEDWomen New Orleans inviting me to talk about my work on the main stage of their international conference. I realized this was a phenomenal opportunity to share my story in a less clinical, statistics-driven way, with a real emphasis on the human narrative.

It took me two months to come up with the story I would tell. Aside from my conversations with the grandmothers, I'd never really spoken about Erica publicly before, but I understood that I would be passing through a new phase in my healing process if I were to acknowledge to a much larger audience that I'd lost a client to suicide. Given that the most successful TED Talks blended personal stories with broader social concerns, I knew that I had a wonderful opportunity to engage a global audience with the work of the Friendship Bench. I hoped to do so in a way that might open people's minds to the power of storytelling in healing larger individual and collective wounds.

I flew into New Orleans and spent several days preparing and rehearsing. I was also pleased to meet a kindred spirit named Leah Chase, the "Queen of Creole Cuisine," who was being interviewed on the TED main stage. At the age of ninety-four, she was still running her restaurant in New Orleans. I was immediately taken by her story of serving her community with soul food and love, and I made a note to visit the famed Dooky Chase's Restaurant, where Leah continued to stir, chop, spoon, baste, and inspire others. I suspect that my immediate affinity for her approach had something to do with the sense of care and welcome that Leah exuded, which reminded me so much of the grandmothers and all the

African women I knew who offered love through their delicious food.

I really had no idea how momentous this trip would prove to be. In many ways, my ignorance of TED saved me. Since I was doing it for the first time and had only recently learned about the opportunity, I was unaware of the potential impact my talk would have. Aside from revolutionizing the art of public speaking, TED has been responsible for launching many passionate advocates into the limelight of international acclaim.

I suspect that had I known all of this in advance, I would have been extremely nervous. But my naivete saved the day. I figured that after my talk, I would have a few days to enjoy New Orleans and soak up the food, music, and people to the best of my ability. I didn't even consider the possibility that millions of people would come to find out about me and the Friendship Bench through that twelve-minute speech.

I was surprisingly calm when the day came to deliver my talk. Two thousand guests populated the auditorium, while another fifty thousand watched the live stream.

When I was finished, I was ready to take a break. After all the preparation and agonizing over the right words and stories to share in a limited amount of time, I was ready for some well-earned relaxation.

I decided to go on a stroll through the city's French Quarter. It was a wonderfully sunny day as I strolled along Bourbon Street, taking in the sights and sounds. Just then, I noticed a sign hanging outside a tiny facade: Marie Laveau's House of Voodoo — All Welcome. I knew that New Orleans was the first multicultural city in the United States, informed by its melting pot of cultures, including those of the enslaved people who were brought to the region and had transported their traditions with them. Still, it was a strange moment; I felt like I was experiencing déjà vu. After my experience in Benin, it was as if I were coming full circle. I took it as an auspicious sign.

With curiosity and eagerness, I entered the cave-like shop. Mystical paraphernalia hung from the walls and ceiling. Feathers, skeletal sculptures, and cauldrons abounded. It was very quiet and cool; I was surprised that nobody else was in this reverential space.

Just then, an elderly White woman emerged from behind a beaded curtain in the back. "Hello, welcome to the temple," she said with a smile.

"As in…voodoo temple?"

She nodded. "Yes! I am a voodoo priestess," she softly replied, motioning me to sit on a small stool in the corner of the room.

I hadn't expected this. "How did you come to be a voodoo priestess?"

"I spent quite a bit of time in Haiti, which is where I was introduced to voodoo. Voodoo liberated me, and since then, my life has become voodoo."

"But you do know that voodoo originated in the African country of Benin, don't you?" I inquired, trying to sound knowledgeable.

"Of course! I lived in Benin for four years after I left Haiti. I was in Ouidah."

"Did you try the pineapples?"

She laughed. "I take it you've been there, too! Amazing pineapples! What brings you to New Orleans?"

I told her that I had just finished giving my talk at the

TED conference. We spent the next thirty minutes discussing voodoo and its essence, which had not changed much over the centuries. Like Mamoudou, she talked about syncretism and how voodoo and the Roman Catholic Church seemed to merge in certain places, especially in Haiti. We also touched on capoeira, a Brazilian martial art that is similar to jujitsu but emerged from slave plantations. It was strange but also quite beautiful to be speaking about these topics with a White American woman who was clearly knowledgeable and had thought very deeply about the core themes and history of her chosen religion. I bought a few items from the shop and thanked her for an enlightening conversation.

"Why don't you join us for a healing ceremony at 5 p.m. if you're free?" she said as I walked out.

"Yes, I'll definitely be back," I replied. I immediately set about looking for a spot to have some good old Southern gumbo. That quest was followed by a series of explorations that led me to so many interesting people and sights that, sadly, by the time I returned to the House of Voodoo later that evening, the ceremony had concluded.

I had been to a number of major cities in the US where I'd interacted with lots of different people of color, particularly African Americans, but what struck me about New Orleans was that the folks here reminded me of home. For the first time, I felt I could connect with Americans in a truly visceral way that didn't require explanation or communication across cultural barriers. Walking down Bourbon Street, I enjoyed my encounters with brothers and sisters making light work of the trumpet, talking Southern cuisine, or sharing their generous spirits in any number of other ways. It didn't really matter what they were doing — all of it felt *grounded*.

Even people who were experiencing poverty seemed to be walking around with a sense of purpose and belonging. Whereas I often felt cautious when I was in a new place, especially when it came to approaching someone to ask for something as simple as directions, I felt deeply connected to the Black people in New Orleans. My sense was that they were rooted in a vibrant, lively ecosystem of cultural and individual connections that made it easy and pleasurable to be among them, despite everything the city had been through over the decades, particularly in the aftermath of Hurricane Katrina.

What I saw was a community with the tenacity to evolve and find new life in the wake of tragedy while never forgetting that it was entrenched in something real, something powerful, something that would always provide a stabilizing bedrock in difficult times.

This was what Grandmother Jack meant when she talked about poverty being a state of mind, I happily thought. *This is how people thrive.*

I got back to Harare on a Wednesday morning.

By this time, I was at the hospital as a university psychiatrist rather than one who was affiliated with the government. My clinical work was exactly the same as it had been before, although I was doing less of it, since teaching and research were taking up a good portion of my time. The blackboard in the admissions ward had fourteen new admissions written on it; I was troubled to see that Resistance was one of them.

I headed back to my car, picked up the day's newspaper, and went back in to find Resistance.

Predictably, he was in the chair where he usually waited for me. He reached for the newspaper and said somberly, "Grandmother Kandawasvika died while you were away."

I nodded, sat down, and allowed a wave of sadness to wash over me. I'd already known that Grandmother Kandawasvika was coming to the end of her road, but the sense of loss always felt fresh every time I received news of a grandmother's death.

I conjectured that Resistance's readmission probably had something to do with Grandmother Kandawasvika's loss, as I remembered that he had also been readmitted in the wake of Grandmother Jack's death. In addition to receiving one-on-one support from Grandmother Kandawasvika, he had continued to come to the peer group that met at the hospital. The Friendship Bench and its offerings had given Resistance a strong sense of a home away from home. He was part of a community of people who were not his biological relatives but who cared for him all the same.

After I sat and talked with Resistance for a while, I thought back to everything that had led to the Friendship Bench. My thoughts naturally returned to Erica and my friendship with her mother, Sekai, which had waned and then faded altogether over the past eleven years or so.

At some point, maybe three years after her initial visit to see me following Erica's death in 2009, Sekai stopped coming to the hospital in Harare. It made me a little wistful to think that our visits were over, but I rationalized my sadness away by coming to the conclusion that Sekai had gone through her own grieving process and didn't need to maintain our friendship, which was perhaps getting in the way of her moving on.

Feeling like I needed my own closure a year after my TED Talk, in 2018 I dug up the notes I'd taken during the time when Erica was my patient to see where she and her family had lived in Mutare. Although I wasn't exactly sure, I knew that a family's name and their ancestral totem often offered clues as to where they hailed from. On the basis of Sekai's surname and totem, I pieced together some additional information about the village where she probably lived. I figured that I would pay a visit to Sekai to say goodbye and express my gratitude for the care and steadfastness she'd displayed in coming to see me all those times. Despite the fact that it had been nearly a decade since we'd last communicated, I hoped that she would welcome my visit and understand that it was my way of offering gratitude. In the wake of the events of the past thirteen years, I felt that I could better articulate how meaningful our friendship had been to me — how it had been an important aspect of my own healing and ability to grieve Erica's death.

I had another good excuse to be there. My maternal grandmother came from a rural community close to Mutare, called Odzi. She also spent half her time in Harare, but in her old age, she preferred to be in her ancestral village. I hatched a plan to take my mother to visit my grandmother and also take the opportunity to see Sekai.

It turned out that I guessed correctly which village Sekai came from. Sadly, however, the people in the area told me that Erica's family had moved away, and nobody knew where they'd gone. I learned that many people in the community had moved to a nearby region where diamonds had been recently discovered — similar to Wenera, the place that Sekai and I had wistfully talked about during our first meeting after Erica's death. It's possible that Sekai and her family moved because they were in search of new opportunities, or perhaps they wished to turn over a new leaf after their daughter's tragic death.

Originally, when I'd hoped to find Sekai, I'd thought about paying a visit to the mango tree that Erica had loved so much and that had been the site of her death. In Zimbabwean culture, after someone takes their own life by hanging themselves from a tree, the family invites a loved one to cut that tree down. I'd wanted to see if the tree was still there, and if I could, in my own symbolic way, cut it down to honor Erica. That intention died as I drove away from the village without having found her family. I recognized and accepted that sometimes closure is a gift only we can offer ourselves.

Now, as I sat in the clinic room after seeing Resistance and considered the trajectory of the past several years, I felt the weight of both the losses and the victories: the many deaths and the many opportunities for celebration. I longed for Erica and Sekai to know how much they'd contributed to my life, and became misty-eyed. It had taken me some time to recognize how important Sekai had been to me and how her gentle insights and willingness to help me through my grief, even in the midst of her own, had contributed to my work with the fourteen grandmothers. She had been almost like an additional grandmother to me. Although I hadn't trained her in the Friendship Bench protocol, our relationship had a quiet intimacy that made me feel like I was talking to a therapist in order to process all that had happened. I had always looked forward to our conversations; being around Sekai made me feel loved and cared for, just like my experience in the voodoo priestess's hut. In a way, we had engaged in a ritual of grief and togetherness in our own community of two.

Through the window my eyes caught sight of the guava tree, as active as ever with its chattering finches. I could still remember how that cheerful sound had filled the room the day I'd met Erica and Sekai; it had often been our soundtrack during subsequent visits. It had seemed to me such a contrast to the nature of the conversations I was having with Erica. But now, as I pondered all that had occurred over the past few years — especially the outpouring of hope that had emerged through the act of community members sharing stories on benches across Harare — I felt a newfound sense of gratitude.

I realized that in the ceremony of life, joy and sorrow often live in close proximity. It was up to us to open our minds and hearts, to cross the bridge between these seemingly opposing experiences and discover that we were not alone after all. Underneath other such trees were many benches and many grandmothers, all of whom were waiting with a smile and a gentle invitation: "Tell me your story, and I'll tell you mine."

Conclusion

In March 2023, almost seventeen years after I met fourteen headstrong elderly women who would change my life forever, the Friendship Bench organization held a commemorative event for the eight surviving grandmothers. It took place at our property, which was five years old and served as a hub for the people in our community.

In addition, a generous Zimbabwean family donated their home, a house valued at over $1 million USD, to the Friendship Bench in 2023. We decided that the old property would become an administrative center and the new one would be where our trainings would take place for anyone who wished to learn the Friendship Bench model. Here, people could come to receive therapy on a drop-in basis and chat with any of the other people on the premises. It was our desire to create an environment where everyone would feel connected on a much larger scale.

For the event, commemorative benches had been affixed with silver plaques that proudly bore the names of the fourteen original grandmothers. This was our way of ensuring their legacy would live on forever, although there was really no symbolic gesture I could think of that was capable of accomplishing such a task. We invited people from all over Harare, as well as funders, government officials, and others who had been among our most enduring allies from the first few bootstrapping years to our current incarnation as a full-fledged NGO.

Although eight of the grandmothers were still alive, only six of them were active, going without fail to their respective benches almost every day. Fortunately, we'd also met the goal that we set so many years earlier: the Friendship Bench was now scaled up throughout all ten provinces of Zimbabwe. Whether someone lived in a city or a rural area, there was a Friendship Bench, along with a wise grandmother, right in their vicinity, ready to provide necessary support.

We gathered together to remark on the changes we'd seen over the preceding years. "You're a whole professor now," Grandmother Kusi joked, "and we're closer to the graveyard!" It was true that many of them were much slower and more frail, cognitively and physically, than they'd ever been, but the fire within them was still palpable. A part of me was convinced that they would be here to offer their wisdom and support to the community of Mbare for many years to come. But another, more pragmatic, part of me — the one who had already mourned the losses of six beloved grandmothers — knew better. Each of the grandmothers was making a gradual but certain progression toward concluding the brilliant and transformative work she'd done in Mbare and beyond. Often, I'd see a grandmother slowly trudging, with measured steps and absolute determination, to her bench — usually with the help of a grandchild, who would return a few hours later to walk her home.

Although I would often see the grandmothers on a weekly basis when I went to visit the hub, it was still a highly emotional experience to be with them, all of us together in one place. It almost mirrored the early years when we'd gather outside the clinic in Mbare, tinged now by the sad fact that we'd lost almost half of the original grandmothers.

Even Nurse Shelly, the mental health nurse who'd had an important supervisory role in the early years of our project, came to partake in the festivities. We all laughed and chatted in the casual, intimate spirit of those who have collectively nurtured a child from infancy into the adolescent years. Indeed, the Friendship Bench *was* the child we'd stewarded from its first wobbly steps and into the current moment, during which new possibilities were continuing to emerge.

My heart was full as I considered that the growth of the Friendship Bench had paralleled my own growth…and that the grandmothers, as well as Erica's mother, had offered me so much compassion as I went through my own grieving process and attempted to harvest a sense of purpose and possibility from it.

Of course, time well spent with the grandmothers would be incomplete without music and dance, and the grandmothers insisted that we all dance together. With the drums accompanying the sounds of laughter and stomping feet, I could feel in my bones that I was participating in a historic moment I would stash away in my memory for years to come. It was very likely the last time some of the grandmothers would dance like this, and the infectious energy of the celebration seemed to reflect the preciousness of the opportunity.

To this day, two of the original five Friendship Benches stand outside the clinic in Mbare, reminding me of our commitment to always maintain benches in places where people live, work, struggle, and thrive. Although community members can come into our new center for therapeutic support or to make a new friend, we will always strive to meet people exactly where they are.

These days, we are proud to be able to offer our Friendship Bench in a Box, a DIY digital toolkit that provides people around the world with all the knowledge we've gained over the many years of doing this work. I continue to receive requests from people across the globe to go to their cities and offer trainings; because we don't have the capacity to meet all the requests, we decided to create something that enables the spirit of the Friendship Bench to take root wherever it is needed.

Although our trainings began face-to-face, in the wake of the 2020 Covid-19 pandemic, they quickly made a transition to a virtual environment, which is how we realized our digital Friendship Bench in a Box could spread like wildfire throughout the world. Today, people in Spain, France, the United States, El Salvador, the Arabic-speaking world, and countries across Africa have received insight into how they can create Friendship Benches in their own communities. And although we strongly encourage the grandmothers in these places to be the primary ones doing the work (they are, after all, our proven gold standard for care and healing), our pool of international implementers includes all kinds of people, young and old. Given the fact that communities and their needs differ widely around the world, we decided that we would not be rigid in the implementation of the Friendship Bench.

For example, in Washington, DC, we have trained grandmothers and grandfathers. In Louisiana, where we are collaborating with the School of Social Work at Southern University at New Orleans, we have an intergenerational group of implementers. In El Salvador, amid a complex brew of social issues that include femicide, poverty, and gang violence, we're working with Catholic nuns, who are seen as go-to resources in their communities.

Through our growth, we continue to learn and to improvise. For one thing, in order to meet diverse communities where they are, we know we need to refine the screening tools that help us to detect whether someone is struggling. In addition, our work in Zanzibar, where we have a strong connection with the Muslim imams and local mosques, led us to realize that religion can be a powerful agent for delivering the Friendship Bench. I had no idea we'd end up interacting with religious leaders (which we're also doing in El Salvador and even in New Orleans), but they often have a strong role to play in stabilizing communities. We must continue to be flexible around our expectations of the Friendship Bench and to let the reality on the ground help us figure out the logistics of how we work (and with whom we work) in any given place. For example, in Kenya, trainees wanted the benches to be placed in the tea estates, because the people who'd most benefit from the model were the ones picking tea. And in New York City, we don't use benches at all; rather, the people helming the Friendship Bench in the Big Apple decided to institute large orange blocks for greater visibility. I was initially worried that nobody would want to sit on such unsightly seats, but I was wrong!

And of course, our work continues to flourish in Zimbabwe, where the intergenerational connection is extremely important. Between 2023 and 2024 in Zimbabwe, over four hundred thousand people sat on a Friendship Bench to share their story with one of our grandmothers. It is these profound and deeply personal stories — of both the clients and the more than three thousand grandmothers we work with — that continue to shape my vision for the future. Stories of pain and hope, like Tamika's, a forty-two-year-old mother of three who lost her family home and assets accumulated over twenty years to her in-laws after her husband's untimely death. With no other place to turn to in her hour of darkness, Tamika visited the nearest bench, where she opened up to Grandmother Rose, one of our newer grandmothers. Tamika shared her harrowing story of rejection, eviction, and destitution. An assault led by her late husband's brothers left her in an emotional wreck and with a high score of eleven on the SSQ, including a yes response to the question of suicidal ideation. Grandma Rose listened compassionately to Tamika's life story of how she had contributed to building the family business, purchasing fixed assets, and paying for school fees for her children. Unfortunately, despite being married for over twenty years, Tamika had no marriage certificate, and none of the family assets were in her name. "We built it together," she lamented. "There was never a need to have anything in my name because it was for the family."

Without judging Tamika, Grandmother Rose leaned into the story with empathy and wisdom. Then, through her resourceful network, in true social prescribing fashion, Grandmother Rose zeroed in on a plan to obtain temporary shelter for Tamika and her children and to engage the local community court over her loss of assets. In addition, Tamika was reassessed by a more senior grandmother to rule out any imminent risk of suicide.

"Opening Tamika's mind took some time because she was overwhelmed by the situation," Grandmother Rose mused as she recalled the sessions. Grandma Rose helped her navigate through the stages of kuvhura pfungwa (opening the mind), kusimudzira (uplifting), and kusimbisa (strengthening), while also being part of a Circle Kubatana Tose community support group and attending at least four court sessions. Finally, after three months, Tamika emerged victorious when the local court granted her legal right to her home, children, and family assets.

Tamika wept uncontrollably as she shared the news with Grandmother Rose and they hugged on a Friendship Bench under a msasa tree. Today, Tamika continues to see Grandma Rose at church in her community, and she is still an active member of her local Circle Kubatana Tose.

As the global population, especially of elderly people, increases, I believe that our world's grandmothers constitute one of our most vital resources. They hold vast wisdom and light, but these can remain sorely underutilized and even unacknowledged in the rush toward progress and in the mechanization of the world. What are at risk of loss are our Indigenous and cultural traditions that center love, care, and the wisdom of our elders.

At the same time, we must also engage the light and wisdom of our younger people, who have much to offer in the way of new ideas and an infectious optimism that has the power to move us in the direction of meaningful innovation.

Although countless social media memes point to the rifts between the generations — with older people blaming younger people for the problems of the world and younger people blaming older people for creating those problems in the first place — our model helps people to see that all of us have wisdom and a perspective that are necessary for the collective.

In Zimbabwe, we currently train university students to become peer counselors, and they are mentored by a group of grandmothers who continue to offer their own services on benches across Harare. It is meant to be a mutually beneficial relationship grounded in a two-way connection of shared wisdom and guidance. The grandmothers provide the younger counselors with best practices (which is part of the benefit of living a long time and recognizing what works and what doesn't!), while the young people help the grandmothers to be more efficient by taking advantage of technology and innovative ideas. Hence, a mutual opening of the minds becomes possible!

Throughout all this work, in both the Global North and the Global South, common themes continue to crop up. We know that no matter where people are located, those with mental health struggles are always dealing with underlying social determinants — adverse childhood experiences, poverty, violence, limited or no access to healthcare, and the list goes on. This is why I often say that the Friendship Bench isn't purely about mental health; it's also about equipping community members to collectively address and heal the challenges they are facing. And with our emphasis on asset-based community development, we can remind people that they have what it takes not just to survive, but to thrive — and to build entire communities that do the same.

No matter where the Friendship Bench goes and how it is offered to communities, I know for sure that one thing will never change: this is a model that is anchored in the power of storytelling to transform us from the inside out.

On that day in March 2023 when I celebrated with the grandmothers and many people who had experienced an awakening in their hearts and an opening in their minds, all because of the Friendship Bench, I couldn't help but think of the wise words often attributed to Maya Angelou: "People will forget what you said, people will forget what you did, but people will never forget how you made them feel."

And it's true. The grandmothers planted a seed of empathy and connection that took root not just in a small community in Mbare but in far-flung places all around the world. All that has flourished in the years after I decided to do something to honor my patient Erica was contained in a simple but profound belief: when you are able to sit next to someone in pain and to maintain the presence and tenderness that help lonely souls remember they are never alone, a ripple effect of healing, beauty, and goodness ensues. Minds open. Broken hearts grow bigger and stronger, creating room for nurturing, empathy, and love. And the seemingly intractable causes of our pain and suffering and of the cycles of violence that threaten to swallow us whole transform. My hope is that we will have the opportunity to experience this wherever we are in the world; so much healing is still needed.

We live at the crossroads of great change, facing circumstances that are asking us to reconsider our disruptive relationship to the natural world and one another. It is clear that the discord we continue to encounter is worsened by a pandemic of alienation and loneliness — by the sense that we are separate islands sitting alone in our own sorrows, rather than interconnected archipelagos of treasures that are waiting to be unlocked in service to one another and the planet.

And now, dear reader, this is where you come in.

If there is anything you've gained from this story of the Friendship Bench, may it be the realization that you need not be a trained professional in order to help others in your community. You don't have to be a cognitive behavioral therapist or a psychiatrist to offer solace to those who are struggling. Every single one of us has the inherent ability to share our stories and to deeply listen to others, especially those who have not traditionally been heard, without judgment. The more we move away from the notion that we must place authority in the hands of "experts" and institutions, the more we will recognize the gifts and strengths that already live within us and all around us, so that we can make a difference with what we have, one story at a time.

Join the Movement

If you are inspired by the Friendship Bench story and you would like to bring a Friendship Bench to your community, school, place of worship, or workplace, you can do so by requesting a Friendship Bench in a Box DIY toolkit. The toolkit guides you through the practical steps of how to set up a Friendship Bench and includes a unique code that gives you access to our virtual technical support team to walk through this journey with you.

Visit www.friendshipbench.org/partnerships and join the movement!

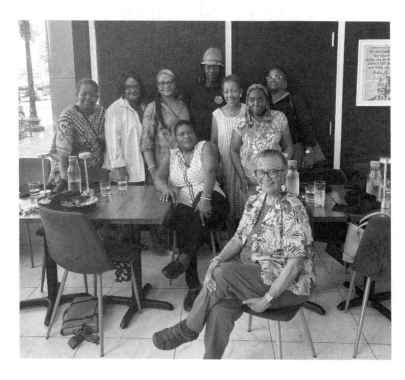

With some of the grandmothers of the Friendship Bench Washington, DC, program in 2024. The time I spent with them as they expanded the program in the Anacostia neighborhood of DC was akin to drinking from a fountain of wisdom and knowledge.

Acknowledgments

I owe a tremendous debt of gratitude to many people who have helped transform the Friendship Bench into a reality, starting with the first fourteen grandmothers, who made it possible for me to see beyond my clinical expertise and truly embrace the concept of *ubuntu* ("I am because we are").

Writing the story of the first fourteen grandmothers has been an emotional journey for me, and I remain indebted to those who have played a part in helping me frame the story as best I could. I am thankful to Sarah Ladipo Manyika, the first person I shared my manuscript with; I believe her initial suggestions on how to render the story more poignantly brought the book closer to what Grandmother Jack and Fred Hickling would have wanted out of my journey.

The beginning of any initiative is often marked by uncertainty and self-doubt, but the wisdom of the late Dr. Sekai Nhiwatiwa, displayed through her gentle probing, led me to think on a bigger scale about the Friendship Bench. It was Dr. Nhiwatiwa who facilitated my initial meetings with the team at King's College London and the London School of Hygiene and Tropical Medicine, a team I have continued to collaborate with for over ten years. I am particularly grateful to Professor Melanie Amna Abas, Professor Ricardo Araya, and Professor Helen Weiss, who were critical in the successful implementation of the first clinical trial of the Friendship Bench, which went on to be published in the *Journal of the American Medical Association*. Although I have become the de facto face of the Friendship Bench project over the years, I am thankful to two dear colleagues, Petra Mesu and Lazarus Kajawu, both clinical psychologists, who played a pivotal role in shaping our first training program, which informed the clinical trial. Training has always been a key feature of our work, and Dr. Ruth Verhey's contribution to the training and support of the junior psychologists and counselors after our first clinical trial has left a legacy of continued peer learning at the Friendship Bench project. Frances Cowan made it possible for me to complete my PhD, which focused on the Friendship Bench, as my local supervisor in Zimbabwe together with Crick Lund as my primary supervisor at the University of Cape Town; beyond that, she consistently made herself available to listen and give her honest opinion about the hardships of academia and research as the Friendship Bench initiative was growing.

I'm thankful to Pam Roy for supporting the journey of this manuscript through her numerous resources and contacts, but above all for her ability to immediately see the big picture of the Friendship Bench and become a trusted custodian of its values, even as we think of expanding in the United States.

Nirmala Nataraj's nuanced insights on how to intersperse the Friendship Bench journey with touchpoints that truly reflected my personal transformation were critical to coming up with a final draft that I felt comfortable showing to my agent, Barbara Moulton.

Ultimately, however, it's the people who have allowed me to share pieces of their stories in this book that I would like to acknowledge. To all of them, I say: Thank you for letting me into your lives.

About the Author

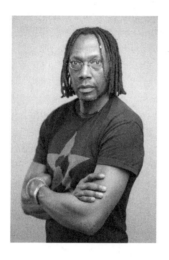

Dixon Chibanda is a medical doctor and practicing psychiatrist with a background in public health. He is a professor of psychiatry and global mental health at the London School of Hygiene and Tropical Medicine and the University of Zimbabwe. He lives in Harare, Zimbabwe, where he spends most of his time overseeing the implementation of Friendship Benches across the country by more than three thousand grandmothers. He also leads the expansion of the Friendship Bench initiative outside of Zimbabwe through a scale strategy called the Friendship Bench in a Box. He has discussed his work with the Friendship Bench in speaking engagements across the globe, and his TED Talk on the topic has had over three million views.